**Double-Feature by Eva Beleco:**

******

# How to Get Rid of Acne and Spots

Successful remedies for blackheads,
rosacea and skin blemishes

******

# The natural Approach
# to Beauty

Tips and recipes for natural beauty secrets -
how to keep your skin and body beautiful
and healthy without chemistry

# About

How to Get Rid of Acne and Spots +
The natural Approach to Beauty
by Eva Beleco




**Copyright and Terms of Use**




**Eva Beleco** is a half german, half australian scientist, whose main interest is a healthy way of living esp. when it comes to chemistry-free cosmetics and beauty-treatments.

# Content

**FIRST BOOK**

******

# How to Get Rid of Acne and Spots

## Successful remedies for blackheads, rosacea and skin blemishes

******

# Introduction

Acne is often seen as an annoying but temporary affliction predominantly suffered by male teenagers. Euphemistically referring to blocked pores as "blackheads" should not distract from the fact that some types of acne are classified as serious illnesses and inflammatory processes in the body.

Some of the more serious types also frequently lead to scarring.

The most common type of acne that is caused by hormone changes in puberty and therefore disappears even without treatment when maturity is reached around the age of 20, is a so-called endogenous syndrome, in other words: a disease pattern caused by the body itself.

This is also true for acne caused by metabolic imbalances at a later stage in life – as an endogenous disease pattern it will disappear along with the underlying problem.

Considered a lot more serious are exogenous types of acne that can lead to the formation of fistulas or lumps and are very difficult to diagnose in terms of their origin. There seems to be a direct correlation between the disease pattern and physical condition and life style of the patient. As a consequence, an improvement of the condition can in most cases only be achieved through life-style changes.

Many external remedies don't bring the hoped-for relief but tend to have the opposite effect instead – especially if they trigger allergic reactions, for example, that aggravate the condition.

For these reasons it can be very difficult indeed to get rid of acne, spots and blackheads. Most acne sufferers have made the discovery that simply buying a new "miracle ointment" is an expensive but ineffective option. So what is Plan B? Try alternative treatment methods or get a prescription for Roaccutan from your dermatologist?

People who don't know what suffering from acne is like often belittle the problem. After all, there are other illnesses that are far more serious or even life-threatening. It might well be true that people with a chronic condition or even an incurable illness would much prefer to have acne instead. However this doesn't mean that this skin condition should be taken lightly.

**Understanding how acne affects people**
Acne can have a very negative impact on the everyday life of those who suffer from it. Those who don't suffer from it should try and imagine the following situation:

Just imagine you had been involved in a road accident which left you with many scratches and cuts, both minor and major, to your face. Cosmetic surgery has hardly made any difference – each time you look into the mirror you have to face those deep cuts and scars in your face.

How would you feel whenever you met people or left your house? Without shadow of a doubt you would feel self-conscious because of those scars and your disfigured face, in particular when dealing with people directly. You think that everybody will recoil in horror when they see your injuries.

People suffering with severe acne feel just like that. They feel disfigured. Every time they look into the mirror they just see their acne – and ignore whatever other qualities they might have. They often feel that other people see them in the same light as they see scarred and disfigured accident victims and are convinced that people just notice their defects and nothing else.

Naturally this is hardly ever the case. As a rule, acne sufferers are much more self-conscious than those surrounding them. But nevertheless the feelings of acne sufferers should be considered a lot more.

**Acne in children**
This is particularly relevant if children or teenagers suffer from acne. Parents think that their children will grow out of their acne phase at some point and ignore their feelings or play them down. After all, teenagers cause a lot of headaches anyway, don't they?

But try to see things from your child's point of view. How would you feel if you were the victim of a road accident and tried to explain to your doctor how much emotional suffering your disfigured face caused you and your doctor didn't take you seriously? Or your partner rolled his eyes each time you mentioned your looks...

Fair enough, most children do grow out of acne at some stage, but even if that's the case – acne is something they have to deal with here and now and that they need help with here and now. Maybe they have to listen to verbal bullying from their class mates on an everyday basis, and without any support from their parents things are a lot worse for them.

**Mild cases of acne can be bad too**
Even mild cases of acne can cause a lot of worries. After all, adolescents want to have a boy-friend or a girl-friend and want to have the perfect looks for them. Even a few minor spots can undermine their confidence.

When you have a date or you are giving a talk in front of your whole class and everybody is looking at you, the last thing you want is spots. If the pressure is on, you just don't want to worry about how to get rid of those unsightly skin irritations.

We often worry a lot about very minor skin blemishes or very small spots – no matter whether other people even notice them or not. Even with a small spot we feel uncomfortable and wonder, if people are going to laugh at us or make fun of our slightly less than perfect appearance.

**What can be done about it?**
In order to get your clear skin back it is important to not just listen to what other people tell you to do, but to find out for yourself what will help to visibly improve your acne. Some people may succeed by using an ordinary spot creme; others might need considerably stronger remedies. In serious cases it is always a good idea to consult a dermatologist. Even then getting a second opinion won't hurt.

If you only suffer from mild acne you might just need a few hints about possible remedies and the right therapy to help yourself. Even more severe types can be controlled without prescription medication. In either case, however, you will have to consider changing your life-style. What you eat can make an enormous difference, no matter how severe your type of acne may be.

In most cases, long-term success can only be guaranteed if you are patient with yourself and give your skin time to heal. Short-term remedies just won't work. Your skin will take a minimum of a month to at least start regenerating itself. Ointments for redness might well show some visible results within a few days, but this doesn't mean you have got rid of your acne once and for all.

**Treatment and Prevention**
Treatment and prevention of acne isn't difficult. There is no need for expensive cremes and lotions or even a doctor's appointment – even though at least in severe cases an appointment with a dermatologist is a good idea. There are many over-the-counter remedies you can get in pharmacies that can help you to improve your skin on a permanent basis.

On the other hand, self-treatment can lead to mistakes that are easily made but make your skin condition a lot worse.

Making your acne disappear is great but it is only half the job done. You want your skin to be fresh and clear looking clean and soft. While some people are born with lovely skin and have to thank their parents and grand-parents for it, others have to work hard to achieve the same. It's just as it is with your body shape. Some people are blessed with a muscular figure and a flat belly while others have to go to the gym, do weight-lifting and watch their diet to achieve the same.

You are not on your own on your quest for the best remedies for a clean and healthy-looking skin. We have talked to many specialists in the field of skin care and we've also done a lot of in-depth research ourselves. In this book we would like to present you with the results of our findings.

**In this book we will tell you the following:**

- explain what causes acne, including myths about hormones, nutrition and the terrible teens.

- openly discuss mistakes you might make looking after your skin and how they can aggravate your acne condition.

- give you advice how to keep an eye on your skin and care for it and by doing that not only alleviate your acne symptoms but also learn how to keep your skin healthy, clean and - even more importantly – well moisturized.

- explain which ingredients are offered by various acne remedies in order to make you understand which ones really work and which ones are useless or even harmful to your skin.


Acne is no laughing matter - neither for children nor for adults. But it doesn't have to be a permanent state. Acne can be treated and disappear for good.

Are you ready to do something about it and live your life without acne? Why don't you have a look and see what we have to say about the topic?

Happy reading!

Best wishes

Eva Baleco

# Getting to know your own skin

Do you know which the biggest organ of your body is? It's your skin, that's right. It really is one big organ with a variety of functions in your body in order to protect it and make sure it stays healthy.

Skin can be presented in a beautiful way (someone putting moisturizer on or rosy baby skin), but there are also a lot of things that can go wrong with skin. Some problems are minor irritations, for example caused by dry skin or minor spots.

But sometimes skin problems can be more severe than just minor irritations. They are not just unsightly but positively painful and even dangerous. One of these problems is acne. And even though most people associate acne mainly with teenagers, adults can be afflicted with the condition at any stage of their lives too.

Before we go into discussing acne and its causes and treatment methods, let's have a closer look at skin in general. A better knowledge of this amazing organ will help us gaining a better understanding of the causes of acne and methods to deal with it.

**Functions of our skin**

Our skin does a lot more than provide good looks and keep our clothes in the right place. Without our skin we wouldn't be able to survive. Let's have a look at the functions our skin has and why it is important to care for it. We will also have a look at problems that can arise.

**Keeping things in place**

Our skin's most obvious function is keeping our organs and intestines in place. The human body is a self-sufficient machine and our skin is vital to keep everything together. In the same way that a car needs bodywork to contain engine, radiator and other parts, our body needs its skin to keep everything in place comparable to a safety net for everything.

This doesn't mean to say that all our inner organs are just randomly scattered in our body. There are muscles, ligaments and sinews attached to our bones and make sure that our organs don't go anywhere. But our skin keeps everything where it should be and stops things from moving. It is the ultimate safety net for everything else.

**Insulation**

Just imagine going out without a coat in freezing conditions or leaving your windows wide open. You will need to keep yourself warm with a jacket in order to maintain your body temperature and not get freezing cold. This is why you have to shut the windows in your house to stop the heat escaping. Your skin is something like a jacket for your body.

Your body produces heat in a similar way to a heater producing heat for your flat. Without your skin the heat would escape from your body in no time at all.

**Protection**

Do you know why cars have windscreens? The answer is obvious. The windscreen provides protection for driver and passengers from anything in the air including dust, insects, dirt etc.

In the same way as a windscreen protects people travelling in the car, your skin protects you from things that you have to face every day – not just insects, dust, dirt, germs and bacteria. Your skin also protects your body from the elements such as sun, wind and rain. It is designed to absorb or deflect these things.

**Pulling force and motion**
Have you ever tried to open a jam jar just after putting creme on your hands? You most likely failed because you couldn't get a firm grip on the jar.

Your skin makes sure that you get a proper grip in order to hold on to things. Although your skin is very soft in principle, it has enough traction force and friction within your clothes and other materials. It stops us sliding off a chair. It allows us to hold things, to sit properly and to stay put.

**The structure of our skin**
All this helps you to understand that the skin is not just a covering for bones and inner organs. If you really want to know how to deal with skin problems, it is a good idea to know about the quality of your skin and, more importantly, what your skin is made of.

Understanding the structure of your skin will give you a better idea of what can go wrong looking after it and how you can get to grips with it.

You don't have to be a dermatologist to understand minor skin problems. Knowing a few basic facts is enough to help you care for your skin in a competent way.

**Skin layers**

Do you know the Greek dessert "Baklava"? It is made with layers of puff pastry that have to be so thin that they look like they might very easily tear.

These sheets are folded over again and again and because they are layered up that way, the final product looks like one single thick layer of pastry – even though it really consists of many ultra-thin parts.

Our skin is structured in a very similar way. Although not folded over, it consists of many different thin layers that combine to give our skin its overall thickness and stability.

It is important to know these different layers in order to understand the problems that can arise and above all which of the layers are responsible for them. That way we are able to get to the root of the problem and take it from there.

There are three principal skin layers: the epidermis - the top layer on the outside – the dermis and the hypodermis.

The epidermis or outer skin layer is remarkable in that it has no blood vessels but relies for nourishment on the capillaries that lie underneath it. This layer is responsible for keeping water in our body and makes sure that no chemicals or other dangerous substances can enter our body. Thus it works as a natural, strong barrier and protects our body from infections.

Underneath the epidermis lies a net-like structure that contains the roots of our hair, sweat glands, nail beds and blood vessels. Many skin problems – including acne – originate from this skin layer.

This may be more than you wanted to know about your skin, but these things are important if you want to avoid skin problems. So-called "stretch-marks" in obese or pregnant women are caused by too much pressure within the blood vessels when the skin is over-stretched. These blood vessels close down which in turn causes the scarring that we call "stretch-marks".

This demonstrates how important it is to know about the structure of your skin and where some of our skin problems and blemishes may come from. We often wonder why ointments and other external remedies won't provide the result we hoped for when we bought them.

This is often due to the fact that these remedies do not penetrate far enough into the skin layers and therefore cannot be expected to work. Taking this into account you are much better able to judge which medications for acne and other skin problems are likely to work.

# Common skin problems

It is probably fair to say that people with perfect skin don't exist. Even photos of the most beautiful models always have to be digitally edited in order to get rid of irregularities, birth marks and similar flaws. Plastic surgeons and dermatologists are always in demand as well when it comes to dealing with skin problems in models and actors.

Knowing more about general flaws of your skin can help you to make a more informed decision how to treat your acne too, as the roots of acne and other skin problems are usually the same. Ideally we won't just get rid of acne that way, but also end up with healthy-looking skin.

**Acne**

Acne is a disorder that takes its origin in the hair follicles in the skin. When these follicles are blocked the pores of our skin get blocked too and show up as spots on the surface at some stage. This blockage and the „bump" signify that there is an accumulation of dirt, talcum, dead cells and other things sealed in that area and this in turn leads to inflammation or unsightly spots.

As I mentioned before, the skin is a living organ that needs blood and oxygen amongst other things in order to stay healthy. In contrast to other organs our skin has to be able to "breathe" which means that it has to get rid of irritations that might prevent that. Blocked hair follicles are neither natural nor healthy which is why our skin reacts with redness and inflammation.

**Blackheads and spots**
Most of us will have seen these minor acne outbreaks in their faces or other parts of their bodies. Before the formation of the bump we call them „blackheads"; after the skin has formed little white swellings on top, we are talking about a spot. These spots are essentially what we define as acne.

In other words, when we treat acne in general, blackheads and spots disappear too.

**Cysts**
Sometimes we confuse acne with cysts, as they can have a similar appearance. Unfortunately cysts tend to be a bit more serious than typical acne.

A cyst is a small enclosed capsule with a separate membrane and partition from the rest of the skin. Cysts can contain air, fluid or other substances.

It is not unusual for cysts to develop not only on our skin but also in the rest of our body. Typically cysts are very small and usually harmless. A lot of cysts disappear on their own accord, but severe cases have to be surgically removed.

In most cases it is not the cyst itself that is dangerous, but rather its position. Cysts in the uterus, for instance, can interfere with a pregnancy. It is up to your doctor to decide whether or not a cyst is dangerous and has to be removed.

**Pigmentation marks**
A pigmentation mark is usually a harmless dark spot on your skin that can occur anywhere. Most people get pigmentation marks within the first two decades of their lives, but some babies are born with them.

A small percentage of pigmentation marks can be malignant, but as a rule it is only an accumulation of cells that contain more pigments than others and therefore appear darker.

Pigmentation marks that change their color or shape can be dangerous and these changes can develop into malignant tumors. Again only a doctor can decide whether or not a pigmentation mark is harmless or needs to be monitored.

## Rosacea

Rosacea is a very uncomfortable skin condition that can easily be confused with acne due to its symptoms such as red and inflamed skin areas.

Rosacea is characterized by:
- Redness of cheeks, nose chin and forehead
- Appearance of small and obvious blood vessels in facial areas
- Minor swellings and spots in facial areas
- Runny or inflamed eyes

Although rosacea cannot be completely cured it can be controlled and at least the symptoms can be alleviated with the right kind of treatment.

In rosacea patients the blood vessels in facial areas expand too frequently and too much. This can be caused, amongst other things, by bacteria or mites. Irritations of the hair follicle, allergic reactions or inflammations of the skin can also be the root of the problem. Other factors are suspects too, but they are still being researched.

It is very important to distinguish between the various causes of rosacea. If people with hyper-sensitive skin get rosacea, treatment with acne products will not be successful but rather aggravate the condition.

For that reason rosacea has to be treated in a completely different way from acne to avoid further damage to the skin.

**Other flaws**

Even though our skin protects us from environmental influence this doesn't mean that it is completely impenetrable and cannot be damaged. Particularly with the progressive thinning of the ozone layer in recent years there has been an alarming increase in skin cancer and other serious skin conditions.

Freckles and so-called "age spots" can often be warning signs indicating damage to the skin caused by the sun. They can also just be due to excessive pigment formation in some skin areas causing spots, irregularities and similar problems.

There are also cases of unexplained tumor growth that doctors have no plausible explanation for. These can occur both on the surface of the skin and underneath the surface. They are not necessarily always cancerous. They can be surgically removed; there are no other treatment methods yet.

Obviously it is vital to go to your doctor if you detect skin growths, especially if they are painful.

# How many types of acne are there?

Acne doesn't equal acne. Before thinking about improving your skin you have to be able to tell the difference between the various types of acne:

**Acne Vulgaris**
This is the most common type and generally known as puberty acne. Apart from a few spots and blackheads in facial and back areas acne vulgaris is usually harmless and doesn't leave any scarring.

**Acne Comedonica**
This type is slightly more serious than acne vulgaris. There are more inflammatory processes leading to small spots. Scarring is not normally a worry with this type either.

**Acne Conglobata**
This severe type of acne causes large pussy pustules that can affect deep layers of skin tissue. Scarring is quite common with this type of acne. Most cases of acne conglobata require medical treatment.

## Acne Papulosa

Is a less severe type of acne that very rarely causes scarring. Nevertheless it is this type that seems to be particularly resilient and can be very difficult to get rid of.

## Acne Papulopustulosa

Severe inflammation penetrates deep into the tissue and leaves noticeable scarring. Whoever suffers from that type of acne should consult a dermatologist. Prescription medication is a must. Luckily this type of acne is very rare.

## Acne Inversa

Acne Inversa is a chronic skin disorder that can occur even a long time after puberty. It involves repeated cycles of pussy inflammation and can in some cases be very painful. Affected areas often expand more and more, so much so that it can even result in restriction of movement.

## Possible acne triggers - and things that don't cause acne even though people think they do

Spots are made up of various substances, for instance sebum, dirt or dead skin cells. Sebum is an important factor for our skin, as it makes sure that it stays soft and pliable. Without it our skin would be as hard as leather. It would often crack and bleed.

Too much sebum in the skin however stops dirt particles and dead skin cells from being removed as they should be. More and more material collects and can't be removed as the top layer of the skin won't open to allow it to pass. When this happens a spot is formed instead.

Under normal circumstances the outer skin layer peals and allows surplus sebum, dirt or dead skin cells to disappear during the morning or evening bath or shower. With skin that is prone to acne, however, sebum and dirt get trapped because the top layer won't allow them to get through.

This explains why a plug is formed, but it doesn't explain why the skin won't allow things to pass through. The answer to this question gets us right to the bottom of the problem we have fighting acne.

## Hormones

If your hormones are out of balance, this can lead to a chain reaction that affects your skin as well. Androgene hormones, for instance, stimulate over-production of sebum. Surplus sebum combines with bacteria and dirt. If this mixture blocks a hair follicle, it can lead to acne.

## Pollution and bacteria

If you live in a very polluted or dusty environment, it is only natural that more of these pollutants settle down on your skin than there would normally be. This can't be helped. But after all it is one of the functions of our skin to protect the body from just those things, so nothing can get into your body. Looking at road workers or miners will show you that their skin has been discolored and looks grey or blackened through constant exposure to dirt and dust. Naturally the pores of their skin can get blocked through this.

**Stress**

Our body reacts to all types of stress and pressure. We can get short of breath or panicky, fed-up, tired or irritable. Many of these reactions can be retraced to primitive physical reflexes to dangers and threats.

It is not clear why our body reacts to stress with acne, but this could be due to an increase in sebum production in times of stress. Our body might feel that it has to protect itself from something. This includes the skin. Increased production of sebum in such a situation might be designed to  better protect our skin.

In any case stress seems to be a trigger for acne, especially in people who are prone to acne anyway. Whatever the reason might be, there is a connection between stress and acne. Therefore you should try to avoid stressful situations.

**Bad eating habits**

A poor diet is poison for our skin and works like a fertilizer for spots and blackheads. Sweets, ready-meals and fast food should therefore be avoided. Try to replace for example sweets by fruit, burgers or pizza by fish, meat, vegetables and rice. Cutting out dairy products can have a positive effect on your skin too, as many people have a more or less pronounced lactose intolerance.

**Excessive cleansing**

In order to protect itself, the body has a few interesting reactions up its sleeve. If for instance you don't drink enough water, your body has the tendency to store water as it isn't getting enough. If you don't follow a healthy diet, your body will get protein and other nutrients out of your muscles, because you aren't providing them.

If you use aggressive face cleansing products too frequently because you think that they help eliminating sebum and bacteria you will achieve exactly the opposite. Your body will react by producing even more sebum to make up for the missing layer. This is a mistake acne patients often make, and it makes matters a lot worse.

**Things that don't cause acne**

It is important to know what causes acne, but it is equally important to know what doesn't. This will stop you trying to use remedies that are not possibly going to work.

**Sweat**

It is hard to believe, but sweat as such doesn't cause acne. It doesn't contain the harmful substances and waste products that people think it does. Sweat is just water that our system brings to the surface of the skin in order to cool down.

The only way sweat can cause acne is when it combines with dirt and bacteria and blocks the pores like that. Sweat itself, however, doesn't contain those bacteria. Therefore it is not a matter of washing it off as soon as possible, especially not if your skin was nice and clean before sweating. As mentioned before, sweat can only cause acne in combination with dirt.

**Cosmetics**

Cosmetics used to be made with ingredients that promoted the development of acne. They contained heavy metals and were often based on oil. The make-up was applied to areas where sebum was trapped and therefore blocked pores very quickly.

Women used to develop acne exactly in those areas where they applied most of the make-up. Why do we still insist that cosmetics hardly ever cause acne? The answer is simple: dermatologists and producers of cosmetics have done a lot of research when they developed their products and tested the effect that different cosmetics can have on our skin.

They have learned to produce better products with better ingredients on a water rather than oil basis, for example.

Water won't block the pores of your skin and won't attract dirt and bacteria. A lot of the ingredients that used to promote spots have been removed from the products. Nowadays practically all products are free from harmful substances.

On the contrary, nowadays most cosmetics are even good for your skin. They contain vitamins such as Vitamin E that helps to moisturize your skin and keeps it supple.

Many doctors even recommend that women with acne use cosmetics as a protective barrier against dust and dirt in the air. As long as make-up gets removed every day, it doesn't cause any skin problems.

**Lack of hygiene**
It is often wrongly assumed that people with acne just don't wash properly, because acne is caused by dirt and bacteria.

Well, everybody has dirt and bacteria on their skin, but not everybody gets acne because of that. Some people are more prone to acne than others, but this doesn't signify bad personal hygiene.

The tendency to develop acne can be due to poor diet or to totally different reasons, but in most cases genetic factors are to be blamed. A greasy skin doesn't indicate poor personal hygiene.

**In a nutshell**
It is important to understand the various factors that can cause acne in order to treat it efficiently. Unless you find out about the source of your own individual case of acne and get the right treatment for it, your acne will always come back.

# Anybody can get acne

Even though it seems to be mainly teenagers who suffer from acne, it is not restricted to teenagers. There is, however, a reason why many teenagers get acne and why in most cases the acne disappears again when adolescence is over.

This happens for the same reason as the one causing many women to suffer from acne around the time of their period or during pregnancy: their hormones "run riot" and have to readjust to changes within the system that happen at the time.

This is independent of sex, as in principle men and women have the same hormones in their bodies – it is the quantities that are different. Women have higher estrogen levels while men have higher testosterone levels.

Hormones influence and control a variety of functions within the system. Causing acne is one of them. Presumably it is a hormone called androgen that is mainly responsible for changes in sebum glands or over-production of sebum. Androgens might be male hormones, but they occur in both sexes. In puberty or during a pregnancy their normal levels can get out of balance.

**Acne in teenagers**

During puberty the juvenile system goes through significant changes, and some of them can take years before things get back to normal. Amongst them are growth spurts, but also various hormone changes and as a result of that a temporary hormone imbalance.

The latter is, of course, a natural part of puberty and the changes affecting the body within that phase. This "hormone crisis" cannot and really should not be interfered with. The body has to sort out by itself which hormone level is right for it and as long as it can manage by itself you shouldn't try to help it along with medication or chemicals.

Nevertheless there are a number of things teenagers should be aware of when it comes to acne and the right treatment of it.

**Cleansing routine**

Cleanliness and tidiness don't tend to be at the top of teenagers' priority list. This applies to their dens and the way they dress, but also to their approach to skin care. Caring for their skin without overdoing it is very important during adolescence. This is why parents should show their children at the beginning of puberty how to clean your skin correctly without putting too much strain on it.

They should be provided with quality products that have a peeling effect, so that dead skin cells can be removed and cannot block hair follicles. A quality moisturizing creme is equally important. All these things are vital for a teenager's skin care.

**Acne in adults**
Many adults know how unpleasant it can be to discover spots on their skin. With most people this is only a temporary skin irritation that fades within a few days. But some adults suffer from spots and blackheads all the time.

It is estimated that around a quarter of all adult men and half of all adult women suffer from skin problems like blackheads, spots or even acne at least once in their lives.

Apart from hormone changes there are various external factors that can trigger acne in adults. The term „cosmetics acne", for instance, describes skin impurities caused by different types of personal hygiene products such as soap, perfumes, wash lotions, shampoos and shower gels, as well as cosmetics.

Drugs and medical products can also lead to acne in some cases. Package leaflets contain information about side-effects of the medication in question and whether it can trigger acne. If this is the case, the producer is legally obliged to point it out specifically.

Equally, a generally unhealthy life-style can trigger an outbreak of acne in adults, for instance a poor diet and lack of exercise. In principle, all the causes of acne in adults are known, but treatment methods have to be individually adjusted to control acne in adults successfully.

A miracle cure for acne in adults doesn't exist. Everybody's system reacts differently to external as well as internal stimuli. For that reason individual acne treatment methods are the key to controlling spots and other skin impurities.

**Acne in women**
Particularly in women, various hormonal changes are seen as the root of adult acne. For instance, many women suffer from spots just before ovulation, but these spots often disappear again at the beginning of the period itself. A blood-test investigating hormone concentration can show whether the patient has a particular tendency to produce certain hormones during that phase.

With some women the transition from adolescence to adult acne is seamless, but with a relatively large number of women the problem appears when they are in their 20's or even 30's. The reason is assumed to lie in hormonal irregularities.

A very common type of acne in women is so-called pre-menstrual acne – the appearance of spots just before the period. The skin irritation starts a few days before the period and goes away at the end of it. Taking vitamin B6 can help to alleviate the symptoms. Women who take the pill suffer less from pre-menstrual acne.

Acne caused by hormones occurs in pregnant women as well as in women during the menopause. In either case the spots disappear again after giving birth respectively after the menopause.

For all types of acne caused by hormones, good personal hygiene as well as an informed choice of suitable cosmetics proves to be successful. Hormone therapy is the last resort when everything else has failed.

**Acne during pregnancy**
Many women report skin problems occurring within the first quarter of their pregnancy. Acne during pregnancy is very common and completely normal because in this phase more androgens are being produced.

These hormones cause an enlargement of the sebaceous glands and therefore increased sebum production. This causes impurities in the skin and leads to the formation of spots.

Please be aware of the fact that not all acne remedies and treatment methods are suitable for pregnant women, even though they are only applied externally. Consulting a doctor is usually only necessary in very serious cases of pregnancy acne.

# Acne scarring

Permanent scarring is only caused by the more serious types of acne, but ordinary spots can leave scars too. This can easily happen if spots are squeezed frequently. If the connective tissue is damaged, new cell tissue is formed that looks different from the ordinary skin appearance.

There are two types of acne scars:

## Hypertrophic scars

Hypertrophic scarring is caused by an over-production of skin cells that close the wound but at the same time leave the affected area with a slight hardening. This over-production of skin cells can be further encouraged by hormonal changes, for instance during puberty.

## Atrophic scars

An atrophic scar is characterized by a contraction of the skin due to a lack of moisture above the affected area where it leaves something that looks like a hole. The skin contraction also leads to hardening of the atrophic scar. First and foremost, however, it is a surplus of melanin that causes this type of scarring through an uneven distribution and gives the top skin the typical scarred appearance.

**Treatment options**

Next to numerous products that promise to make your acne scars disappear but often fail, there are the following dermatological treatment options:

- High concentration fruit acid peelings

- Removal of acne scars by laser treatment

- Microdermabrasion


These treatment methods will be discussed in more detail under the chapter heading: „Acne medication and dermatological treatment methods"

# How to look after your skin the right way

In the context of treatment, control and prevention of acne a good skin care routine is extremely important. By skin care we mean cleansing, moisturizing and nourishing it.

For acne patients proper skin care is particularly important. Regular skin care will not only speed up the healing process, but also reduce the formation of new spots.

Many people with acne tend to put too much strain on their skin by washing too frequently, rubbing too hard when they dry their skin after showering, using the wrong cosmetics products or allowing their skin to get too dry.

Allowing your skin to get very dry is a big mistake. Your system's natural response to dry skin is producing more sebum in order to moisturize the affected areas.

If acne comes about because of too much dirt, sebum and bacteria accumulating and dead cells not getting removed, wouldn't it be a logical conclusion to wash as frequently as possible? But it doesn't work like that. You have to know exactly how and how frequently you should clean your skin, and which products to use to make sure that it stays free from acne and has a healthy appearance.

Let's have a closer look at ways to cleanse your face to help you understand the extent of the problem.

**Over-cleansing and dry skin**

It is important to remove grease from your skin in order to keep it clean. But as we pointed out above, your skin produces its own grease that is needed to keep it healthy and soft. If you clean it too frequently and use products that are aggressive towards your skin these natural oils are removed. This leads to your skin drying out and producing wrinkles.

**Correct cleansing routine**

Cleaning your skin is important to prevent acne and for its treatment; dirt, bacteria, excess sebum, dead skin etc. are removed from the skin's surface. That way, pores and hair follicles cannot be blocked by these substances which in turn would lead to the formation of spots.

Unfortunately too much cleaning or cleaning with aggressive products has a counter-productive effect and can cause skin irritation and thus aggravate your acne.

Regardless how bad your acne is, it is important that you are gentle when you are cleaning facial areas. It is not a good idea to scrub your skin and make it sore when you wash. Mild cleansing products are normally strong enough to remove make-up and dirt.

When you are using lotions or cleansing foam, you should apply them with gentle, circular movements. When using pads or cotton wool, apply the cleansing product very carefully with upwards movements only. This is the best way to get impurities out of your pores.

Your facial cleansing routine should consist of the following steps:

Very little cleansing is necessary in the morning. A gentle face lotion will be sufficient to wash the surplus grease off that has accumulated during the night. There is no need to use soap or very concentrated facial cleansing products.

This should be followed by a moisturizer. Women have to make sure that this is done straight away to allow the moisturizing creme to sink in before make-up is applied. Men should also apply a moisturizer in order to protect their skin from dirt, sweat and grease.

There is no need for additional cleaning during the day unless your work-place is extremely dirty or dusty. If this is the case, you should remove the dirt as soon as you are back home.

The evening is the most important time for facial cleansing. For women this means that they have to remove their make-up completely. After that use a face lotion to protect your pores as they will be open now. After the face lotion has dried you should apply moisturizing creme.

Once or twice weekly (don't do it more frequently) you can do a peeling. Make sure that you always use a moisturizing creme after exfoliating.

## Exfoliating/Peeling

The purpose of exfoliating is to remove the top layer of the skin. This is where all the dead skin cells and other impurities are that make your skin look bad.

There are many products for peeling on the market. You have to bear in mind, though, that exfoliating of the top layer of your skin also removes things your skin needs like sebum and moisture. If you repeat the procedure too many times, your skin can get too dry, in which case you have the additional problem of flaking skin in facial areas.

Exfoliating using face brushes or similar products is much too rough for your skin and therefore not recommendable. Some peeling cremes contain peach stones and other natural ingredients designed to remove the top layer of your skin. They may well be too aggressive for your face. Don't rub too hard, be gentle on your skin. You shouldn't punish your skin for having acne, even if you may sometimes feel like that.

A better choice for a peeling product is mild and water-soluble foam that contains cleansing pellets. Many acne patients make the mistake of exfoliating too frequently. They think they should exfoliate when their skin is dry, in order to get rid of the dead skin. However, it is much better to get to the root of your dry skin problem rather than resorting to constant exfoliating.

**Different types of peeling**
Cleaning your skin down to the pores every now and then can be a very pleasant experience – particularly if you suffer from greasy skin. Fruit acid peelings, for example, are even good for scars. The following types of peelings are available:

**Classic Peeling**
Traditional peeling involves small particles that have an abrasive effect and rub off dead skin particles.

This type of skin peeling is not recommended with acne, as it breaks down the skin's natural protective layer and generally doesn't achieve an improvement.

**Fruit acid peeling**
Slightly more suitable for acne patients are fruit acid peelings. Fruit acids or glycol acid penetrate the top layer of the skin particularly easily due to their small molecules and encourage a removal of the horny skin from the inside.

Fruit acids for cosmetic purposes exist in different concentrations, usually between 5% and 40%. Higher concentrations of more than 30%, however, are only used by dermatologists for the treatment of acne scars.

For private use only products with a maximum of 15% concentration are suitable. After treatment with glycol acid the skin is red and irritated. Therefore fruit acid peelings should not be used more frequently than once a month.

**Salicylic acid peelings**
Salicylic acid peelings are the best for acne. Salicylic acid not only causes the skin to peel, but also prevents the formation of new spots by counteracting the bacteria that cause spots. If you don't overdo it,

this ingredient can definitely improve the appearance of your skin.

**Moisturizing your skin**
If you suffer from acne, because your skin is too oily, why would you keep your skin moisturized?

As soon as you deprive your skin of the important natural skin oils it has a tendency to over-compensate by simply producing more. In other words, the more and the more frequently you remove oils respectively sebum from your facial areas, the more your skin is going to produce.

This is why it is so important to put moisture back after cleaning your skin. By the way, his does not only apply to acne skin but to normal dry skin as well.

The choice of the product that you use and which ingredients it contains plays an important part. Initially try Vitamin E oil. One tube usually costs less than 10 Euros, it does not cause any irritation in sensitive skin and women can even use it in the morning under their make-up.

**Cosmetics and acne**
The option to cover up spots with make-up is very popular with women who have skin problems. But many cosmetics contain ingredients that actually

promote acne and people who don't read the list of ingredients can considerably deteriorate.

Unfortunately even 'oil-free' cosmetics that don't come with an acne warning are unsuitable for acne skin. They too can block pores and promote the formation of spots. For that reason you should do without make-up if you can. If you are unsure about what to choose, ask your doctor or your pharmacist.

A valid alternative to make-up is a sulphurous powder for a light cover that also prevents acne. Sulphur has anti-bacterial properties, but also makes the skin dry. Therefore it is more suitable for people with oily skin.

Important points:

Remove your make-up thoroughly and make sure that there are no left-overs.

Don't use too much make-up. Allow your skin some ‚breathing-space‘.

Only use products that are suitable for your particular skin type.

# Cleansing and facial care products

In the past the only product people used for washing was soap. Washing lotions and cremes for sensitive facial skin were developed much later.

But even today you shouldn't use cheap shampoos, peelings or soaps if you can avoid it, as they irritate the skin and damage its protective layer.
It can be difficult to find the right cleansing and skin care products, partly because there are so many of them to choose from and all of them promise the same things.

As certain cleansing products are not only of no benefit to your skin but can also cause it considerable harm, you should have a good look at the ingredients of a product before you allow it to get on your skin.

Don't be fooled by the details given such as the pH-value. It goes without saying that the pH-value has to be around 5.5, but this is no guarantee that the product is suitable for acne skin.

Equally, products containing alcohol are to be used with caution, as they dry your skin out. Alcohol may not be bad for your skin in general, as it is very good when it comes to dissolving grease, but there are better ways of removing dirt and oil from your skin.

So next time you purchase shampoo, deodorants, hair spray, make-up or other cosmetics, find out first if they might aggravate your acne. If possible, buy these products from a pharmacy or buy natural cosmetics as these are tested for ingredients, efficiency and harmful substances as well.

We recommend products that not only moisturize your skin but also reduce redness and help you skin regenerate.

## Soap

Many people still use soap to wash their face. Unfortunately cleaning agents that are suitable for your hands are not great if you apply them to your face as they tend to be far too strong.

Most types of soap contain extremely aggressive ingredients that- if used for that purpose - practically remove all natural oils from the skin. Without those natural oils, however, your skin dries out.

A feeling of tightness and ultimately more wrinkles can be the result. Apart from that most soaps contain perfumes and other additives that can harm the skin in facial areas. Perfumes and colorants in particular can be extremely irritating for your facial skin.

With this in mind you can use soap for all parts of your body where the skin is not sensitive, but soap should never be used for cleaning your face, as it dries the skin too much.

**Face wash**

Face wash was invented in ancient Greece where a mixture of animal fats, bees' wax and water was used to soften the skin. It was only in the 1950's and 60's that face wash became popular in this country – at first by women who used it to remove make-up. As mentioned before, back then make-up used to be a lot more harmful to the skin than it is nowadays.

When purchasing face wash for sensitive skin you should pay particular attention to the following points:

They should be water-soluble which means that they can be completely rinsed off with water and leave no residue at all. Avoid products with added perfumes. Anything you use should be free of perfumes and additives. Your face wash should also be soap-free as soap dries the skin.

**Face toners**

Face toners can be very good for your face. They help to close the pores after you have just washed your face or applied a face mask. They also absorb excess sebum and moisturize your skin when it gets too dry. Mainly people with greasy skin or with skin that is prone to acne should use face toners. They can help moisturizing your skin after washing without depriving it of natural oils.

**Face masks**

Face masks are recommended to a lot of people who are prone to acne because of their anti-bacterial properties and their ability to remove both bacteria and dirt from the skin. The top layer of the skin is peeled off while the skin is being moisturized at the same time. There are face masks that can do all this, but you have to be very particular when you try them out. Here are some points you have to consider when you make your choice:

Avoid face masks that contain anti-acne ingredients, as a high concentration of these ingredients dry your skin and act as an irritant. The skin areas around your cheeks and eyes are the most sensitive areas in your face. These areas should not get into contact with your skin mask that should only be applied to your forehead, nose and chin.

It is vital that you always apply moisturizing creme after a face mask. Most masks make your skin dry even though they contain a moisturizer as well.

**Special acne products**
What about special acne skin cleaners? Shouldn't they be perfect as they are formulated for acne skin? Unfortunately that's not the case. Many acne cleansing lotions contain a concentration of benzoyl peroxide that helps to remove excess sebum and kills bacteria that cause acne. The problem is that these lotions are applied to the entire face and not just problem areas.

Ironically, it is often products that are especially designed for acne sufferers that are the worst thing you can do to your skin. With a high concentration of anti-acne ingredients they are likely to dry your skin and cause even more irritation which can lead to further acne episodes.

The same is true for medical products. We tend to see them as the best solution for our problems. But the problem with „proper" acne medication is the fact that these remedies contain a lot of alcohol or acetone that merely dry your skin and can also cause redness, flaking and a stinging pain. Your face can become sensitive to pressure and develop even more acne problems.

**Astringents**
As the name indicates, an astringent is a substance that causes the skin to contract. It is the effect caused by tannine in some types of fruit that makes your mouth go funny. An astringent applied to your skin causes the blood-vessels to contract. This makes the skin appear harder.

Acne patients are often told to use astringents to make their skin look drier and appear less greasy. But the only thing astringents actually do is remove the natural oils from the skin, they don't treat acne. The skin might get drier, but this is more of a disadvantage than an advantage. One thing is for certain, your acne won't get cured this way.

**Organic and natural products**
Many peoples' skin is sensitive to chemicals. Therefore products with natural ingredients like camomile or aloe vera are often a better choice.

**Ingredients you should look out for**
Not only moisturizing cremes but all skin care products should contain natural ingredients and oils. Vitamins A, C and E are very important for healthy skin and should always be part of the ingredients. Other natural ingredients are:

## Coconut propyl betaine

Coconut propyl betaine helps through its natural moisture content to prevent the skin from losing its natural oils. Furthermore it doesn't clog up the pores or follicles and allows the skin to „breathe".

## Vegetable glycerine

Vegetable glycerine attracts moisture and makes sure that it stays within the skin without blocking the pores. It is made from vegetables.

## Camomile

Camomile has naturally antiseptic properties that help dry skin to heal. Many doctors have confirmed the beneficial properties of camomile for the skin. Even just tea-bags with camomile tea placed on red or swollen skin areas help to soothe these symptoms.

## Walnut shell extract

Walnut shell extract is a mild antiseptic and a natural remedy that helps to remove dead skin particles.

## Fennel extract

Fennel has a very soothing effect on the skin. The extract has antiseptic properties that benefit sensitive skin.

Peppermint oil

Peppermint oil is refreshing and has a moisturizing effect. It helps to relax the skin and can be used to treat muscular pain and cramps.

Hop extract

Hop extract acts as a toner for the face and enhances blood circulation. It also has a soothing effect on skin irritations and helps to get rid of redness, swelling and other disorders affecting the surface of the skin.

Olive tree leaf extract

Olive oil is very good for your skin. Not only does it provide moisture but also has anti-inflammatory and anti-bacterial properties. Olive tree leaf extract works as a natural moisturizer without irritating your skin.

Fruit extracts

Juice and extracts from fruit are ideal for sensitive skin in facial areas.

Yarrow extract

Yarrow enhances blood-circulation which in turn helps the skin to heal itself. It is often recommended for sensitive skin.

<u>Mistletoe extract</u>

Mistletoe extract has mild and subtly antiseptic properties that are particularly suitable for oily skin.

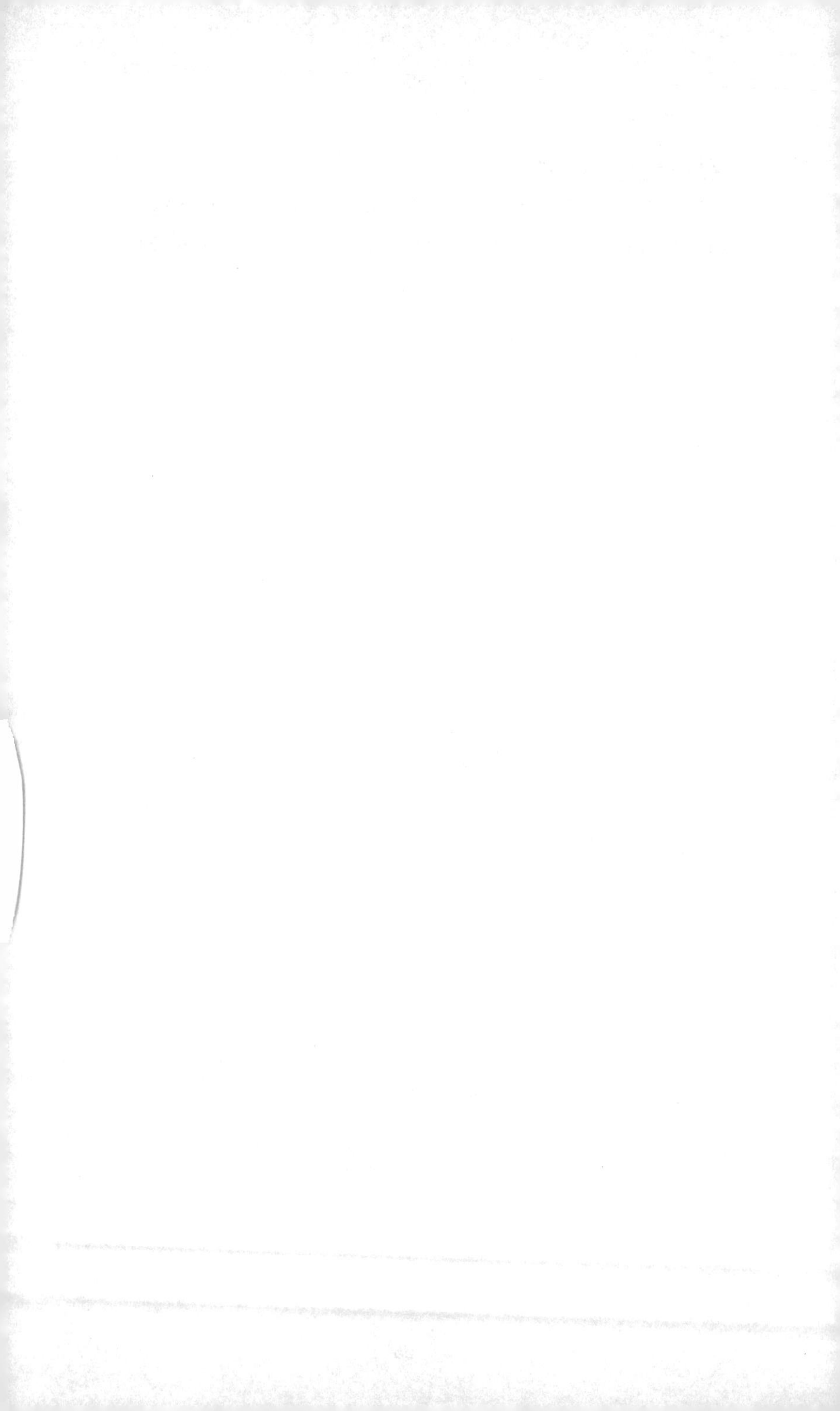

# How to make your own cleansing products and face masks

Using cleansers with natural ingredients is probably the best thing you can do for your skin. Natural ingredients irritate your skin far less than strong chemicals. It isn't difficult to make facial cleansers and masks with natural ingredients at home if you know what to put in and how to use them.

Here are some simple recipes — especially made for skin prone to acne or for oily skin in general. If any of the suggested mixtures cause any problems, stop using them immediately. Although most mixtures are very mild and can't really cause any problems, each skin type reacts differently.

**Simple face cleaner and peeling mask**
Mix half a tea-spoon of baking powder with half a cup of water and add a bit of peroxide. The mix should be a thick paste. Adjust the amounts of water and baking powder accordingly.

Don't add too much peroxide — a few drops are enough. Apply the paste to your face, allow it to dry and leave it on for a while. Rinse thoroughly with cold water.

## Simple egg mask

Eggs are rich in protein, Vitamin A and fatty acids, all of which are very good for your skin. You can just use a raw egg, whisk it and apply it to your skin with a cotton wool wad, or you can first add a little oil containing Vitamin E. Leave the mask to dry for about 15 minutes, then rinse off with cold water. This simple but effective face treatment can be used once a week to hydrate your skin and moisturize it.

## Honey and oatmeal mask

This is probably one of the oldest mixtures ever used when it comes to home-made facial cleaners. Simply mix honey and oatmeal to combine it into a sticky paste. Apply it to your face and leave it to work for 15 minutes. The oatmeal absorbs excess sebum and dirt and helps to moisturize your skin. This mixture can also be used as a peeling mask if you massage it into your skin with circular movements. Do this for several minutes and rinse with cold water.

## Tomato mask for greasy skin

Peel the skin off the quarter of a tomato and press through a sieve to remove the pips. Add two table-spoons of natural yogurt, two or three slices of pu-reed cucumber, one quarter cup of oatmeal, two teaspoons of Vitamin-E-oil and one crushed leaf of mint.

Mix the ingredients well and apply the paste to your face. Leave it for ten minutes, then remove gently by using a flannel with hot water.

## Yogurt and honey mask

This combination has also proved to be very popular for many years. Just mix equal parts of natural yogurt (not fat-free or fat-reduced) at room temperature with slightly (!) heated liquid honey. Apply the mixture to your face, leave it to dry and remove gently with a flannel and hot water.

## Magnesium hydroxide mask

Simple magnesium hydroxide is ideal for use in face masks. Apply a thin layer to your face and leave to work for 15 minutes. Then rinse with cold water. This mask is an excellent remedy for greasy skin.

## Lemon and strawberry for greasy skin

Lemons and strawberries work as a natural astringent for greasy skin. Combine a tea-spoon of lemon juice with two egg-whites, a few tea-spoons of warm honey and a cup of strawberries. Mash the strawberries and add them to the mixture. Apply the mask to your face and leave to work for ten minutes. Then remove by gently dabbing with a flannel and hot water.

**General advice for use**

As a rule, people prone to acne and greasy skin also have a very sensitive skin. Although the suggested masks and face cleansers are made with natural ingredients, they can cause redness and stinging. This is a lot less likely to happen than it would be with chemical products.

It is a good idea to start off with a very mild variety of a mask (don't apply the whole lot straight away) and only leave it on for a few minutes. When you have done a test run and things are going well, you can go on to using recommended quantities and treatment times.

If there is any discomfort or you feel that the mask isn't good for your skin, stop the treatment and try something else. Even natural masks should not be applied more than once to twice a week.

Please bear in mind: if something works in low respectively correct strength, it doesn't necessarily follow that more of it would be even better. Keep to the recipe when mixing the ingredients and don't exceed the application times either.

**Don't forget:**
Home-made masks and face cleansers contain no preservatives and therefore only keep for a limited period of time. To play safe, only prepare what you need for each individual treatment. It is not a good idea to save anything for later applications.

# How diet and daily exercise can influence your acne

Are you tired of being told that you should mind what you eat, drink a lot of water and take as much exercise as possible? Most of us admit that they are. But if you suffer from acne or other skin problems you should listen to this kind of advice.

Let's have a closer look at the correlation between diet, exercise and healthy skin.

**Your diet and your skin**
Whenever you eat something, your food is broken down into its basic particles and these chemical elements are absorbed by your digestive system. Within your body these elements are taken in your bloodstream to where they are needed. Calcium, for instance, goes to bones and teeth, water molecules to each one of your body cells and so on. Waste materials are discarded when you go to the toilet.

Almost everything we eat is processed by our system and gets used for something. Proteins and amino acids, amongst others, are distributed throughout our body and get to our skin as well.

This also means that too much oil or fat we consume is passed on to the skin as well. Whilst some fat is good for us and helps to keep the skin soft and supple, too much fried or deep-fried food leaves surplus fat in your system and on your skin as well.

Nutrition is not only a very widely discussed topic; it is also fraught with many misunderstandings and myths. It is certainly true that acne can be considerably improved and you can even get rid of your spots completely if you eat a healthy diet. Therefore it is worth trying to find out about ways to achieve this.

Some people dismiss the point about the influence of diet on acne by arguing that "acne is caused by hormones, not by what you eat" – or: "I know people who eat junk-food all the time and they don't have acne." It is fairly obvious where that line of reasoning comes from – it is people who would love to get rid of their acne but are not prepared to change their eating habits.

People with that philosophy are probably going to keep their acne for quite a while yet. It is a fact that a healthy diet provides a good protection against spots and acne. It works equally well during puberty as it does for adult acne sufferers.

The problem does not lie in the question whether or not things work but how they are achieved and maintained. If you really want to improve your acne, you will have to do much more than just go without sweets and dairy products.

**Popular myths**
One of the most popular myths ever must be that fat is bad for you in general. This is quite simply wrong, it all depends what type of fat you consume.

A further myth based on the first one is that in principle vegetable fats are good for you and animal fats are not. This is often maintained by vegetarians who are eager to bring across the third myth that „meat is bad for you". There is nothing wrong with a vegetarian life-style, of course, as in view of factory farming and the quality of meat nowadays "meatlessness" is certainly a good approach. But as far as acne is concerned, a diet containing meat cannot be rejected on principle.

There is no perfect guideline for a healthy diet. Everybody is different and in the same way the needs of each body regarding food differ from each other. For this reason you have to develop some kind of "sixth sense" for things that are good for your body and things that are not.

**Some (almost) always valid guidelines:**

Firstly it is fair to say that unprocessed food is better than processed food. Therefore it is better not to eat fast food, tinned food or ready meals or at least have them as little as possible. Chances are that you will notice a vast improvement in your acne just by doing that.

Another thing that seems to be successful with many people is cutting out dairy products for a month. This has helped many acne patients to become almost spot-free.

Equally you should try to avoid foods with a high content of polyunsaturated fatty acids and get the balance right between Omega-3 and Omega-6 fatty acids.

Even cutting out foods that are rich in carbohydrates as bread, pasta, cake, rice and potatoes has achieved positive results with some acne sufferers. It is up to you to try if it helps.

"Low Carb" diet has established itself and is well-known by now. The only problem is that it is often misinterpreted and misapplied. Just the fact that something might not contain carbohydrates doesn't mean it is good for your health.

As a rule, before you attempt to turn your diet up-side down it is a good idea to consult a dietician. They will establish what nutrition type you are and provide you with a tailor-made diet plan.

This is definitely money well-spent.

Good things you can still eat when you have a prob-lem skin
If junk food has a negative effect on our skin it is only logical to assume that nutritious food has a positive effect. And this is actually the case. If we eat well our skin looks good.

Vitamins, minerals and fatty acids are vital for our skin in order to look healthy. They help many parts of the body to repair themselves and to get rid of dead cells. A lack of these important vital nutrients will become obvious, and not just in the shape of bad skin.

We are often told that fruit and vegetables are good for our health. They contain all the important nutri-ents that we need for our health in general and for a healthy skin in particular.

Although most types of fruit and vegetables apart from very few exceptions have a positive effect on our skin, the types with a higher concentration of

Vitamin A, C and E are the most beneficial ones. The following types of fruit and vegetables are the ones you should eat as often as you can:

-Oranges and other citric fruits
-Apples, bananas, peaches, plums etc.
-All types of berries
-Tomatoes
-Green leaf vegetables, including all kinds of lettuce. In particular dark green types are good for you, such as spinach and cabbage.

**Important exception:**
This doesn't apply, if you are allergic to one of the foods mentioned above. In that case this type of food is NOT suitable for you in particular.

**What you drink makes a big difference**
We are most probably not telling you anything new when we say that your body consists mainly of water. When there isn't enough water in your system it will show sooner or later. Your skin will be affected as well, and get a dry and wrinkly appearance.

If you think that you drink enough, have a good look at what it is that you drink on a daily basis. As drinking coffee, tea and lemonade is not the same as drinking water. Caffeine for instance has a diuretic effect, which means you are more likely to lose than gain water through drinking coffee. Drink sufficient water — that's the answer. As a rule you should drink at least one liter, better two, over the day. This amount can vary drastically according to life style or eating habits. If in doubt, consult a dietician. If you find water doesn't appeal to you, add a bit of fruit juice or try fruit- or herbal teas.

Try different types of water and, if possible, always take a bottle of your favorite water with you. Regular fluid intake is a matter of habit.

**Controversies about good or bad nutrition**
Over the last years there have been arguments about which types of foods could trigger acne. Studies have shown that not everyone who eats chocolate, fatty and deep-fried foods necessarily gets acne.

On the other hand it has been demonstrated that acne sufferers dramatically improve when they change their diet and cut very fatty food out. While it is debatable whether or not some foods can cause or promote acne, there is no doubt about the fact that vitamins and minerals are important for all aspects of your health including that of your skin. Therefore there is no excuse for not eating a healthy diet.

**Vital substances and nutritional supplements**
In the same way as your entire body needs vital nutrients in order to stay healthy, so does your skin. The most important ones are vitamins and minerals.

Ideally they should be eaten as part of a healthy and balanced diet, but they can also be taken as dietary supplement that can make up for deficiencies in vital nutrients.

Taking supplements is not necessarily recommended and should only be done to support a healthy diet.

**Zinc**
Zinc is one of the best-known supplements for acne patients. Most of them will have used it in the shape of tablets or ointment.

It is indeed a fact that zinc treatment makes a visible difference very quickly, as it accelerates cell growth within the skin and plays an important part in supporting our immune system.

Unfortunately zinc deficiency is wide-spread nowadays, which is due to food processing on the one hand and on the other hand unhealthy eating habits many people have.

## Vitamin C

Our body needs Vitamin C for countless procedures, such as activating the immune system, building connective tissue and regenerating the skin. Acne patients who take Vitamin C often find that their skin has improved within only a few days and feel a lot fitter and healthier in themselves.

## Vitamin B5

It might not be 100% proven that Vitamin B5 is a remedy for acne and spots, but many acne patients swear by a high dose of Vitamin B5 just the same and report astonishing results.

## Biotin

Biotin not only helps with brittle hair but also with impure skin. It supports our metabolism with the digestion of carbohydrates.

## Niacin

People with a niacin deficiency often suffer with red spots and dry and chapped skin. In the shape of Nicotinamid, niacin can be used for external acne treatment too.

## Special combination remedy for acne patients

Recently a "miracle pill" has been advertised that supposedly contains all important ingredients to cure acne. In most cases these tablets are merely vitamin products with a combination of zinc, biotin and other nutrients – the only difference being the fact that they are vastly over-priced.

Most acne sufferers are therefore better off buying important nutrients such as zinc, biotin and Vitamin B5 straight from their pharmacy.

**Physical activities and healthy skin**
Exercise and sport bring many advantages, one of them being better and purer skin. But where is the connection between exercise and a healthy skin? Let us have a brief look at the way that exercise influences our body.

<u>Better blood circulation</u>
Our heart is constantly pumping blood through our system, and the more frequently our heart beats the more blood is pumped around our body.

Our blood circulation has several functions within our body. Blood cells carry vital nutrients that can reach the places where they are needed that way. Our skin, for instance, needs these nutrients.

When we exercise, our blood is pumped through our bodies more frequently and more nutrients get to their destinations in the system.

Another important function of the blood is the removal of waste products. Blood cells not only deliver vital nutrients, but also get rid of dead cells and various toxic substances.

With an increased blood circulation during exercise and sport our body benefits as a whole and more waste products can be removed that would otherwise accumulate in our skin amongst other places. As a result, our skin as a whole appears healthier and purer.

Most people with a regular exercise regime will notice that the appearance of their skin improves and that they look healthier altogether. Better blood circulation is one of the crucial reasons for that.

Another important factor for healthy skin is oxygen. Our skin needs oxygen molecules in order to look healthy and to purify itself. Oxygen too is carried in our bloodstream and taken to the relevant places.

We can therefore achieve an enormous improvement regarding our skin when we exercise regularly. Physical exercise is good for our entire body, not only for our skin.

# Acne medication and dermatological treatment methods

If you have followed the advice given so far, and you have even adjusted your diet, you should be able to notice visible signs of success in your battle with acne. If you still suffer from spots your acne is serious and leaves you with two alternatives:

Treatment performed by a doctor, dermatologist or at least professional beauticians. There are, for instance, treatment methods like microdermabrasion, laser treatment, some types of skin peeling and prescription medication, of course. In this chapter we will try to discuss some of these methods and medication options and enable you to make an informed choice.

Alternative treatment methods such as various exotic oils, homoeopathic options or Traditional Chinese Medicine (TCM). These options will be explained in the following chapter.

As to date acne as a medical condition has not been fully investigated yet, finding the right medication is often difficult and has to be adjusted to each individual case.

Due to the complexity of the condition and its origin (parthenogenesis) a dermatologist should be consulted for severe acne cases and advertisements by the pharmaceutical industry ignored. But even specialists don't always get it right.

**Antibiotics**

Prescribing antibiotics for acne is a very drastic measure that adversely affects the general state of health as they can have considerable side-effects and long-term effects. Nevertheless antibiotics are still being prescribed as medication for acne.

But is this type of medication actually a good idea? Normally oral medication such as tablets has a far stronger effect than antibiotics in the shape of ointments, cremes or gels that are applied externally to the affected areas.

Therefore antibiotics in tablet form are given to patients with severe acne in particular. They have an anti-inflammatory effect and are designed to fight acne bacteria from the inside. They do not prevent the formation of blackheads, but can stop blackheads getting inflamed in some cases.

Simultaneous treatment with a peeling product that helps minimize the development of blackheads is therefore a good idea. Orally taken antibiotics get into the bloodstream and are taken straight to the inflamed follicles. Thus they become active exactly where they are needed.

Medication with antibiotics should be restricted to the most severe cases of acne, if prescribed at all and under no circumstances be used in a long-term therapy. In the long run antibiotics stop working and are very likely to encourage resistances to form.

Furthermore, as part of a long-term therapy the active ingredients in the tablets can have a negative effect on the gut flora which can lead to fungal infections. In many cases the spots return anyway as soon as the patient stops taking antibiotics.

Despite these side-effects oral antibiotics can be useful in severe acne cases. This aggressive approach can make sense for patients with severe acne episodes and achieve almost instant relief and quick improvement. A positive influence on scarring has also been observed. If antibiotics are only used in severe cases and in combination with other acne remedies, the result can be a considerable improvement in the appearance of the skin.

But even then oral antibiotics should only be taken as a temporary measure. The duration of the treatment has to be decided by the doctor. You should never just stop taking antibiotics. Even if there is no apparent improvement, only the doctor in charge can decide what is to be done.

In the case of topical application (antibiotic cremes etc.) the patient should avoid exposure to direct sunlight as the skin can react in a hyper-sensitive way.

Conclusion:
Antibiotics are not an ideal remedy to be used in long-term acne therapy. In the long run they damage the immune system and should therefore only be used in extremely severe cases.

**Roaccutan/Isotretinoin**
This medication may be very effective, but it has considerable side-effects; for that reason dermatologists only prescribe it in very severe cases of acne.

Products containing Isotretinoin (13-cis-retinoic acid) have been the „secret weapon" since the 1980's. Marketed by the Swiss company La Roche in 1982, they are now available as generic drugs as well. Well-known brands are Accutane (USA) respectively Roaccutan. The effectiveness of Roaccutan respectively the active ingredient Isotretinoin is indisputable.

By reducing the production of sebum, spots are sensibly or completely reduced too. This effect comes at the cost of considerable side-effects, though.

The majority of possible side-effects affects the skin itself. Not only the outer skin but also the mucous membranes dry out. This leads almost always to secondary symptoms such as flaking, dry lips, nose bleeds, eye infections etc.

The skin becomes vulnerable, heals very slowly and is prone to scarring, even after the smallest of scratches. If dryness of the eyes occurs it can restrict your ability to drive – especially driving at night can be a problem.

A number of additional side-effects – some of them occurring with a probability of up to 30% - have been observed, that don't always or exclusively have to be caused by Isotretinoin: elevated liver values caused by disturbances in the lipid metabolism, Vitamin A intolerance, painful muscles and joints, possible interference with contraceptives, inflammation of the kidneys, nervous disorders, mental disorders (depressions), and many more.

<u>Conclusion:</u>
Roaccutan can be a successful remedy for acne and is effective in preventing spots. It also reduces secondary skin inflammation caused by scratching, for instance. It is a prescription medication and should only be taken when recommended and monitored by a dermatologist.

**Laser treatment**
Laser treatment is only advisable in cases of mild to moderate acne. Treating acne with laser is still controversial, as there are studies on the subject that are in parts contradictory.

Nevertheless many patients report that their laser treatment has been very successful. As a matter of fact laser reduces the number of those bacteria on your skin that are responsible for acne and stimulates the skin to produce more collagen.

At a price of several hundred Euros per treatment, however, laser is the most expensive option to get rid of your acne. In most cases several sessions are needed to achieve a permanent improvement.

In addition laser treatment can have side-effects, even if advertisements show the opposite. The most common side-effects are redness of the skin (similar

to sunburn), itchiness and small blue dots on the affected areas. All these symptoms however disappear again relatively quickly.

**Photo therapy**
Photo therapy fights bacteria that clog up pores or
hair follicles and cause infections there. These bacteria are killed off during the treatment. Photo therapy is increasingly popular as a treatment of acne
and acne scarring. It is reputedly effective and kind
to the skin.

**Laser- and photo therapy for acne scarring**
Laser-and photo therapy are both suitable for the
treatment of acne scarring, as they work on the top
skin layers and make sure that less or no scarring occurs when spots heal and new tissue grows.

As a rule, photo therapy is safer and more comfort-
able than laser treatment that is more invasive. Be-
low find a list of some of the most popular types of
photo therapy:

Blue light exposes the skin to a very weak source of
blue light that destroys bacteria. Blue light therapy
is not painful, but it has to be repeated as soon as
new bacteria have developed. There can be reactions like slight redness of the skin and drier skin
than usual after treatment.

Pulsating light and heat are used in combination to „damage" sebaceous glands to reduce sebum production.

Laser diodes also affect the sebaceous glands within the middle layer of the skin without damaging the skin surface layers.
Cosmetic treatment options
Chemical peeling and dermabrasion techniques are treatment methods that require more expertise and therefore have to be performed by dermatologists or professional beauticians.

With so-called chemical peelings an active agent is applied to the face that removes parts of the top-layer of the skin when it is peeled off again to reveal the layer of healthy skin underneath.

This treatment method has been applied for many years to counteract wrinkles, laughter lines and sun damage as well as minor scars or acne, of course. After the treatment the skin takes a certain time to recover, but as a rule chemical peelings – if performed correctly – are routine procedures that are tolerated well.

Dermabrasion is mainly used in cases of significant scarring. A rotating steel brush removes the top layer of the skin where scarring is as a rule. Derm-abrasion can be unpleasant for the patient and in general it takes a bit longer until the skin has completely healed after treatment. As laser- and photo therapy are much kinder to your skin, they are the ones that people tend to go for as a rule.

**Microdermabrasion**

Mikrodermabrasion works in a similar way as derm-abrasion, but instead of a steel brush there is a device that shoots tiny aluminum particles at the skin. This way the skin is virtually polished. A mini vacuum cleaner then removes the crystals and along with them dead skin particles. Part of the top layer of the skin is removed in the procedure, and existing scars can be considerably reduced in size.

Skin abrasion can treat acne scars, birth marks as well as wrinkles. Superficial problems respond particularly well. Beauticians sometimes use a gentle variety of the procedure before skin peelings.

<u>The procedure</u>

As a rule a local anesthetic is applied to the skin area to be treated first of all. Then the top layers of the skin including scars are removed with a so-called „polisher". After that an ointment is applied to the skin together with a bandage if necessary.

The treatment lasts between 30 and 120 minutes, depending on the size of the skin area. As skin continually renews itself the procedure has to be repeated several times in some cases.

<u>Mikrodermabrasion and the risks involved</u>
If not enough of the affected skin layers is taken off the result is not satisfactory as there are remnants of scars that haven't been removed – even if they are less obvious than before.

If too much tissue is removed this can lead to disorders within deeper tissue layers through renewed scarring or to redness of the skin. There must be no acute inflammation of acne scars, as they can spread to surrounding skin areas. Equally, microdermabrasion must not be used with skin diseases such as neurodermatitis, psoriasis or acne rosacea.

<u>Nota bene</u>
Do not drink any alcohol after treatment, as it has a blood-thinning effect and can cause complications because of that. You shouldn't smoke either after treatment because smoking considerably slows the wound-healing process down. Exposure to direct sunlight should also be avoided.

<u>Prices and costs</u>

Microdermabrasions can be obtained in hospitals, from dermatologists, beauticians and specialized beauty salons. Before any kind of treatment a dermatologist should be consulted, so potential risks can be highlighted.

Costs vary considerably depending on where you go. As a rule, your health insurance won't cover the costs, so you will have to pay for yourself. Depending on the treatment, costs per session vary between 50 and 100 Euros.

**Choose what's right for you**

Admittedly, some of the treatments described above sound rather invasive and like they could be rather unpleasant. On top of that there are often side-effects such as redness, swellings and so on, although as a rule they quickly disappear again with the right kind of ointment.

Any dermatologist can give you advice regarding the best methods for your individual type and severity of acne. As this kind of treatment is usually not covered by your health insurance, it is a good idea to get in contact with your insurance and ask your doctor for a quote before you start treatment.

At the end of the day you have to decide if one of the treatment methods discussed above or indeed one that your doctor might have suggested is right for you. When you have your preliminary appointment with your doctor, make sure you include the following questions:

- What results can you reasonably expect from the treatment? It is very rare for the skin to recover completely, but visual improvements are always achieved (which helps to reduce distress levels in the patient).
- Will the treatment have to be repeated, and if that's the case, how often?
- Will the treatment make sure that there won't be any recurrence of acne?
- What side-effects are to be expected and how long will they last? Is it going to be painful and if so, what kind of pain-relief can you get?
- Will you have to take time off work or adjust you daily/weekly routine in any way?
- How experienced is the doctor with this kind of treatment? Is there any documentation you could look at or ratings by other patients?
- Are your expectations realistic or do you hope for too much?

All the responses you will get have to be carefully considered before the decision is made.

**WHICH acne products?**

Any pharmacy will be likely to have an entire area reserved for acne products. They range from homoeopathic remedies to medical lotions and ointments for external use. How can you tell which of them are going to work for you and which ones might even make your acne worse?

Many manufacturers promise impossible things like „Get rid of your spots overnight" or „Instant cure" etc. These promises are of course impossible to keep. Even a dermatologist would not be able to make you spotless within just a few days. Many people invest thousands of euros in acne remedies over the years without any real success. Before you purchase just any old product, make sure you find out about the ingredients first and whether the product is suitable for you.

It is vital that you understand which main ingredients are used in acne medication in order to make the best choice for yourself.

Some products work by killing the bacteria that cause acne. Others are designed to remove excess sebum from the skin and make sure that dead skin particles are taken away instead of blocking the normal sebum flow. Then there are products that try to combine two or more of these targets.

## Benzoyl peroxide

Benzoyl peroxide is a very potent ingredient, strong enough to get rid of some acne varieties. However, it has been known to affect areas that are only slightly or not at all infected with acne and cause redness of skin in these areas. It is therefore important to restrict the use of this product to the affected areas only in order to avoid the negative effects on the rest of your skin. Benzoyl peroxide combines two functions: it kills bacteria around the infected area and removes excess sebum.

As a rule benzoyl peroxide is available in different concentrations ranging from 2.5% to 10%. It is not unusual for benzoyl peroxide to irritate the skin by causing redness and even minor swellings in the areas where it is applied. As it also removes protective sebum the skin can become more sensitive to sunlight, increasing the risk of getting sunburn.

## Salicylic acid

You don't have to be a chemist to know that a product with "acid" in its name must be relatively strong and can harm the skin if used by people who don't follow instructions. Many acne products contain salicylic acid, as it slows down the peeling of the skin within hair follicles.

Similar to benzoyl peroxide, salicylic acid is available in different percentage proportions. If you use a product with salicylic acid it is a good idea to start with a weak concentration, as redness and irritation of the skin can occur for the same reason.

As your skin will be more sensitive to sunlight you should always use sufficient sun lotion when you are exposed to it after using salicylic acid.

**Glycolic acid**
Glycolic acid removes dead skin particles from the top layer of the skin and has also got an excellent peeling effect. The ingredients penetrate a long way into the skin – all the way down to the hair follicles, and make it possible to work immediately at the point where acne develops.

Glycolic acid is sometimes added to combinations containing salicylic acid in order to make it reach the deepest skin layers. If glycolic acid is used too frequently this can lead to premature ageing of the skin and cause dryness, redness and skin irritation.

**Sulphur and Resorcinole**
Sulphur and resocinole are rarely used individually, but are usually found as a combination in acne products. They work by removing dead skin particles and excess sebum. They are very effective products that

can break up spots and blackheads. They also frequently cause redness, flaking, stinging and nausea for several days. For that reason they should be used very sparingly.

## Alcohol

Alcohol dehydrates the skin and should therefore be avoided if possible. If you read the list of ingredients on the labels of acne products you will find alcohol in some form in most of them. Many manufacturers add alcohol to their products to remove excess grease from the skin. However in most cases these products are so strong that they do more harm than good and should therefore not be used.

## Acetone

Acetone works in a similar way to alcohol. It removes excess grease but at the same time natural sebum that the skin needs to stay supple. It is a very strong ingredient and therefore not used in many acne products. If you do have to use it, apply as little as possible.

## How to use these products

Being aware of the effects that the individual ingredients can have on your skin will help you to decide which remedies are most suitable for you and how to avoid harming or even damaging your skin.

Whenever you use an acne product you should apply it sparingly and only on the real problem areas. Never apply them to the whole of your face because you think it might prevent acne.

Your cheeks and the area around eyes and mouth are very sensitive and should generally be excluded from acne treatment – unless, of course, they are affected by acne too. With problems in those areas you should however not use aggressive products but stick with mild remedies.

It is advisable to use acne products only once daily. The evening is the best time, just before going to bed, as you skin repairs itself during the night. Especially women should do it that way, as acne remedies are in general not suitable as a foundation for make-up.

If your skin reacts with redness, inflammation or itchiness to any acne product you have applied, either discontinue the treatment or at least reduce frequency of application.

# Alternative treatments

Alongside the conventional treatment methods discussed above there is a variety of alternative methods – ranging from traditional homeopathy to different exotic oils and traditional Chinese medicine (TCM).

**Homeopathy – the body heals itself**
Traditional homeopathy is probably the most popular alternative to conventional medicine within Europe. Many conventional doctors still doubt the value of homeopathy; as in recent years homeopathy has proved to be very effective in fighting diseases, there is now, apart from so-called homeopathic practitioners, an increasing number of doctors who at least partially integrate homeopathic methods in their treatment spectrum.

Traditional homeopathy as a concept goes back to Samuel Hahnemann. It is based on a 200-year-old therapy form that hardly interferes with medical issues. Traditional homeopathy is geared towards the total picture of symptoms in a patient, which requires specialized knowledge and long-term treatment.

Homeopathic treatment methods exercise a powerful attraction. In the past, great healers have achieved sensational success with homeopathic medicine. Amounts can vary enormously and are tailored to the picture of symptoms and the general state of health of the patient. It is a gentle and individual way to guide the patient back to health.

**Homeopathic acne therapy**

Apart from many different ways of administering plant-based active ingredients that can be prescribed in a variety of doses in the shape of tinctures, ointments, powders or globules, there is a number of other methods that are also classified as homeopathic.

One of them is treatment with benzoyl peroxide that releases oxygen in glands blocked by sebum. By releasing oxygen in the glands blocked by sebum, sebum production is reduced and bacteria are killed off. This remedy is available in your pharmacy as gel, suspension, creme or lotion.

Marigold (calendula) makes the skin supple and removes calluses. It has antibiotic and anti-inflammatory properties. In acne therapy calendula tincture in a 1:3 mixture with water is used to dab on the skin three times a day.

Particularly for the initial stages of acne many practitioners recommend a compress made with oatmeal and vinegar. Oatmeal and cider vinegar are mixed in a 2:1 proportion and stirred into a paste. This paste is applied to the affected skin area that is then steamed for 20 minutes with a hot cloth. Vinegar draws the germs out of the skin and oatmeal has a soothing effect.

**Manuka oil**

Based on tradition as well as modern scientific research, manuka oil is regarded as a tried and tested remedy for a variety of disorders. It is extracted from wild manuka plants that grow in New Zealand. Manuka leaves are long, narrow and acicular. They have a strong, aromatic smell and an attractive bitter taste.

The plant has been known since 1769 when James Cook arrived in New Zealand. His crew used manuka leaves to make tea. The plant was used for healing purposes a long time before that, though, as New Zealand's first inhabitants already knew its healing properties and used it to treat burns or inflammations, for example.

Manuka plants contain many valuable medical ingredients such as leptospermone, triterpene acids, ellagic acid and esters. Interestingly, all of them are lipophilic, which means they are soluble in fatty substances. Due to this property the oil derived from the manuka plant dissolves well in clusters of bacteria that cause acne and exercise its healing influence there.

Furthermore, some of its components evaporate very slowly, and as a result the oil adheres extremely well to surfaces and can thus be absorbed by the skin. Manuka oil is surprisingly active and extremely effective in comparison to other aromatic oils of a similar kind.

Manuka oil is an ideal acne remedy. It can be used to make cremes, shampoos, soap etc. All available cosmetics products with manuka oil are particularly suitable for cleansing the skin if you suffer from acne. To date, no adverse effect have been reported.

**Tea tree oil**
Tea tree oil is a surprisingly effective natural remedy derived from the bark of the Australian tea tree and is used for a variety of skin disorders. Its healing properties are due to essential substances, the main ingredient Terpines-4-ol has a disinfecting and soothing effect at the same time.

Although at first sight it seems to be quite an unremarkable product, it is astonishing how many people have improved their condition by using it.

Visible improvement can be noticed after 3-8 days of tea tree treatment. The skin has lost its redness and has fewer spots. The pores contract and sebum production is reduced. When most spots have disappeared the treatment can be applied less frequently.

The oil is simply applied to the affected areas with a cotton wool pad and not washed off, if possible. Ideally clean your face thoroughly before going to bed at night, apply the oil and leave it to work over night. In the morning your skin will feel soft and smooth.

Important:
When choosing the product try to make sure that the tea tree oil has exclusively been made for application to the skin. If that is the case, the terpines-4-ol content is particularly high and there is no risk of contamination.

**Jojoba oil**
The jojoba bush has seeds that look like nuts and are harvested for different purposes. Inside the seeds there is wax that turns liquid at room temperature –

this is jojoba oil. Although we call it „oil", its consistency is not comparable to that of ordinary oil. The wax from jojoba seeds is of very high quality and is used for cosmetic as well as industrial purposes.

Jojoba wax contains valuable vitamins such as Vitamin A and E and also a very positive fat composition. Due to these properties the oil can provide very intensive care for the skin and is suitable for almost all skin types. As it isn't really an oil at all, it doesn't leave an oily residue on the skin, sinks in very quickly and provides sufficient moisture.

Because of its many positive qualities jojoba is seen by many acne sufferers as a „miracle drug". Many of those who are cured swear by the healing power of various jojoba products. The oil has anti-inflammatory properties and is also very soothing.

It regenerates the skin, helps with growing new skin cells and has a very faint but pleasant odor. Furthermore it has a natural 3-4 sun protection factor.

Particularly for acne treatment there are various products such as cremes, lotions, bath essences or soaps that contain jojoba. There are also special face masks that are enriched with jojoba oil. If a cosmetic product has no jojoba oil in it, it can easily be added. A few drops are sufficient for a powerful effect.

<u>Make your own jojoba mask for acne skin:</u>
Jojoba masks for acne and other skin conditions are very easy to make. Just use the pulp of a cucumber or an avocado and apply it to your skin mixed with a few drops of jojoba oil.

You can also use undiluted oil; just sprinkle a few drops on your index finger and rub into the affected area. Jojoba is very skin-friendly and doesn't cause any irritation at all. There are no known side-effects to date.

**Cajeput oil**
Cajeput oil is obtained through steam distilling leaves and smaller twigs of the cajeput tree. Its healing effect has been known for many centuries. In contrast to other essential oils it is not only used in alternative medicine, but in traditional medicine as well.

As a remedy for acne the oil from the cajeput tree can be applied in different ways. One of them is washing the skin in a mild concentration, ideally without using a flannel. Another option is adding it to bath essences, it is also often found as an ingredient in cremes, lotions or soaps. Using the oil for aromatherapy is another possibility; a fragrance lamp, for instance, can spread the oil scent in the room without leaving any residue on your skin.

All essential oils can cause allergies. Therefore it is a good idea to talk to your doctor or homeopathic practitioner before you start treatment.

**Kanuka oil**

Kanuka oil is obtained from the leaves of Kanuka trees. As it is closely related to the Manuka tree, the Kanuka tree is often referred to as "white Manuka". The oil has to be steam-distilled from leaves of the tree.

The original inhabitants of New Zealand already knew about the healing and soothing effect of the ingredients. They brewed tea with the leaves or rubbed Kanuka oil on wounds and inflamed skin.
The oil is a traditional remedy with a scent of herbs and earth that works as a pain-killer, kills germs and helps with rheumatism and inflammations. Due to its cortisone-like virtue it is also used for muscle pain. Other areas of application are allergic reactions, allergic skin conditions, and treatment of respiratory diseases and with acne.

The essential oil has a similar effect as tea tree oil. It can also be used for itchy or irritated skin as well as acne. For the production of cremes, lotions, ointments, soaps or bath essences Kanuka oil is combined with other essential oils, such as black cumin oil, manuka oil or aloe vera. The combination of active ingredients achieves an even better effect on the skin.

As Kanuka oil is a very mild remedy that is mainly used in combination with other essential oils, there are no known side-effects or risks. The oil also has an antihistamine component.

**Propolis**
Propolis is a so-called cement resin, that is produced by bees and serves mainly to make the bee-hive waterproof. To obtain it bees collect resin from the flower buds and barks of trees, preferably poplars, willows and aspen trees.

Propolis contains a variety of highly effective healing substances including essential oils, numerous vitamins and minerals as well as organic secondary plant compounds.

Due to its numerous active ingredients propolis can be used for a variety of diseases – both internally as externally. Internally the resin is a remedy for angina, asthma, bladder infection, bronchitis, gout, flu or cardiac arrhythmia. Externally the active ingredient is used as a remedy for eczema, verrucas, abscesses, athletes' foot, ulcers, shingles, herpes, corns and acne.

For acne treatment for instance a tincture made from propolis powder or granules can be applied. However, caution is required as propolis tinctures are very powerful.

It is also possible to wash with a diluted tincture or add them to a bath. For that purpose the tincture has to be diluted with water to soften the effect on the skin. Diluted tinctures can also be used to apply to the skin with a brush.

Propolis tincture compresses can also be applied to affected skin areas. As an alternative there are different propolis cremes, shower gels, shampoos or body lotions, all of them available in pharmacies and drug stores.

Propolis resin can trigger allergic reactions. It is now a well-known fact that allergies to the active ingredients are not uncommon. It is safe to say that people with known allergies to peru balsam, cinnamon bark, poplar shoots products or caffeic acid should not go for propolis treatment.

Some people might also experience cross-allergies with composite plants. In most cases they are a delayed allergy, which means that symptoms don't become apparent immediately, but during the course of the treatment. It is therefore recommended to speak to a doctor before starting a course of propolis treatment and get some tests done to exclude allergic reactions.

## Mud therapy – a veritable wonder drug

Healing mud is available in form of a powder that has been obtained from loess deposits from the ice-age. It is used for the treatment of numerous diseases – both internal and external.

The healing mud powder has to be mixed with water, mixed well and either applied externally or taken internally. The most important ingredients are oxygen, calcium. aluminum, potassium, iron and silicon. It also contains negligible amounts of magnesium, hydrogen, titanium and natrium.

Even during the modern era healing clay was used as a healing remedy. Later Sebastian Kneipp amongst other people made it famous.

Healing clay can be used as a remedy for all kinds of symptoms, for example for inflammations, neuro-dermatitis, varicose veins, contusions and bruises or rheumatism. It is most popular for use against acne, though. Numerous products containing healing clay are available in pharmacies and drug stores. Healing clay can also be used in pure form.

The way it works is very simple: the cooling effect caused by the healing clay narrows the blood vessels. As the clay dries on the skin, it produces a sucking effect extracting excess lipids and tissue fluid from the skin. These liquids are channeled to the outside. At the same time the interior tissue is heated up and stimulates the metabolism and the blood circulation.

The powder is available in pure form or ready to use. Pure powder has to be mixed with water and stirred into a thick paste. This paste is applied to the face where it has to be left till it has dried completely respectively no dark patches are visible anymore. For that reason, don't apply it too thickly as it could take a very long time to dry. Used as acne treatment it has to be applied twice weekly.

There are no known risks or side-effects with healing clay therapy.

**Traditional Chinese Medicine**
Traditional Chinese medicine (TCM) has always been interested in investigating acne. According to TMC-philosophy the main cause for acne lies, in the same way as it does in the case of other dermatological problems, in an accumulation of interior pathogenic temperature.

This temperature rises – as all heat naturally does – upwards to the head and the upper region of the back where it causes acne.

In traditional Chinese medicine dermatologists make a connection between the affected skin areas and particular inner organs that are affected by a disorder as well. Acne in the area of forehead and nose, for instance, suggests a disorder of the lung, spots and pimples around the mouth one of the stomach. If there is acne on chin and neck, TCM assumes liver problems.

If there are spots with pus, there is, according to TCM, an accumulation of negative fluids in the body, also described as „phlegm in the body".

TCM also mentions the particular case of acne in women. This type of acne gets worse during the period, accompanied by period pains and changes within the monthly cycle. According to TMC this is due to stagnation of Qi and blood in the liver.

<u>Note:</u>
Qi is seen as general vital energy or spiritual energy in TCM. The principle aim of TMC is to restore the natural balance of the Qi in the body. (Source: de.wikipedia.org)

For the cure of acne TCM applies the method of Chinese Phytotherapy. Medication has to be tailored to the individual patient and has to be taken for two to four months. The prescriptions usually consist of Chinese medicinal drugs that are designed to restore the body to harmony within itself.

As a supplement to the medical treatment acupuncture is used in certain cases. The duration of the therapy depends on the severity of the illness and can last between two and five months. In most cases, first signs of improvement occur after the first month.

# The twelve worst mistakes you can make with acne

There are many options to choose from to prevent acne or to fight it — however there are at least as many things that can make it worse. The following chapter deals with the 12 mistakes that are the worst you can make in our opinion when you suffer from acne, spots and impure skin.

**1.  Squeezing spots (the wrong way)**
When you squeeze spots you damage your tissue and make your skin even more vulnerable to infections. For that reason you are better off leaving the job to a beautician or else purchase a comedo squeezer.

As a lot of people won't leave their spots alone, we have collated some important bits of information about how to deal with spots the right way.

- Before you start you should soften your skin. The best way to do that is a camomile steam bath. It helps to open up the pores and the spots can be removed with a lot less pressure.

- Now you can try to pull the skin around the spot away from it. If this doesn't do the trick you can exercise gentle pressure to express the spot. If it refuses to budge leave it alone until the next day.

This is what you shouldn't do:
There is an option to spear the spot with a sterile needle. We don't recommend this method, though, because it can do a lot more harm than good if it isn't done right. The same applies to syphoning the spot with a syringe.

## 2. Not enough hygiene

If you are in the habit of touching your face with dirty hands, change your pillow case very rarely or allow greasy hair to hang into your face, you create an ideal environment for spots and blackheads.

Washing your face should be part of your daily routine in the same way as brushing your teeth is. Don't wash your face just once a day or even every other day – but regularly and at least twice daily. Removing the dirt from your face that accumulates during the day is extremely important. Only then can you expect to get healthy skin and keep it too.

If you do this regularly and follow the other pieces of care advice in this book as well, you vastly improve your chances to get rid of your acne for good.

## 3. Too much hygiene

It is however true that you can do too much in the way of personal hygiene. If you wash your face four times a day possibly even using aggressive cleansers each time, if you apply disinfecting spray to each spot the minute it emerges, you don't do your skin any favors. Skin takes time to regenerate itself.

Even the mildest cleansers will remove important oils and moisture from your skin. They are not the same fatty substances causing your spots. Your skin needs natural oils in order to stay healthy and supple. If your system registers that your skin lacks oils, it automatically starts producing more. This is why it keeps happening that too much hygiene can provoke more acne.

Solution: Make a habit out of a balanced washing routine as suggested in this book.

## 4. Not enough Moisturizers

Men in particular can be reluctant to use a moisturizing creme, as they think it is "unmanly".

But the same rule applies to women and men: if your skin's natural moisture is out of balance and you do nothing about it, you will not only have more problems with impure skin but also get more wrinkles than you normally would.

The best moisturizers contain natural ingredients like vitamins and herbs. The most expensive ones aren't always the best, though; some of the reasonably priced ones are surprisingly good. The products should ideally be water-based, not oil-based (except for Vitamin E oil, of course).

## 5. Cheap products

Most products sold in supermarkets are bad news for acne patients. They are often produced at extremely low cost and benefit mainly the producers, whereas those plagued with spots don't get what they hoped for. Products available in pharmacies respectively from producers of natural cosmetics are usually much better, even if these high-quality products are slightly more pricy.

The same applies to cheap make-up. Earlier on in this book we mentioned that make-up does not necessarily cause acne, but it is still better to avoid cheap make-up.

Even though nowadays make-ups don't contain ingredients any more that clog up pores and many types are actually very good for your skin, this is unfortunately not true for all makes and brands. Some of them still contain ingredients that can clog up pores. The following you should be aware of and make a point of avoiding them:

- Talcum
- Glitter
- Perfume
- Titanium
- Wax
- Zinc
- Formaldehyde
- Propylene glycole
- Glycerin
- Parabens

Cheap make-up tends to contain the above ingredients because higher-quality ingredients are expensive, of course. As this is not always the case and lower range make-up can contain good ingredients you will have to check the ingredients carefully before you buy a make-up brand for the first time.

## 6. Using too many products

It is more than likely that mixing too many acne remedies will only irritate your skin and aggravate your acne. This doesn't only apply to cremes and lotions, but in particular to acne cleansing products, moisturizers and skin peeling products.

Solution: Find *one* mild cleansing product for sensitive skin and with natural ingredients, *one* moisturizer or Vitamin E oil and *one* acne product (if any at all). If you use several at the same time your skin will dry out and it will also lead to increased sebum production.

## 7. Junk Food

Bad nutrition is poison for the skin and works like fertilizer for spots and blackheads. Ready meals and fast food should be avoided as much as possible. Try for instance to replace sweets by fruit, burgers or pizza by fish, meat, vegetables and rice. Cutting out dairy products can have a very positive effect on the appearance of your skin, as many people have a more or less developed sensitivity to cows' milk products.

## 8. Lack of determination

If you want to get rid of your spots you can't do it in a half-hearted manner and give up with the next acne episode. It is rather a long-term commitment and you'll have to give it your best.

When you have decided which treatment or which product you want to go for, you should be consistent and stick with it for a while. The desired success is usually delayed in most cases. Exception to the rule, of course, is when the product doesn't agree with you or there are severe side-effects.

## 9. Lack of sleep

When you don't sleep enough your body lacks this vital time it needs to recharge its batteries and will not stay healthy in the long run. This applies to the skin as well, of course. It too benefits from sleep because it can regenerate itself during that time. Why don't you give it a go? You will be amazed how much difference sufficient „beauty sleep" will make.

## 10. Nicotine, alcohol and drugs

Stimulants and drugs virtually make spots and acne blossom. If you have a problem with acne you should therefore stay clear of alcohol, cigarettes and most certainly hard drugs.

## 11. Not enough liquids

Your body needs water amongst other things in order to eliminate toxins from the system. When you take in enough fluids, the blood-circulation in your skin will be much better and toxins are taken away.

<u>Important:</u> Try to drink water or unsweetened herbal- or fruit teas and avoid dehydrating drinks like soft drinks, lemonade, coke, coffee, tea esc. (a rule that doesn't just apply to acne sufferers).

## 12. Bad mood

They say that "your skin is the mirror of your soul". People who are constantly stressed and bad-tempered often look like it — stressed and bad-tempered. Try and look on the bright side of life. Make a conscious effort to smile for a whole day. Take a proper break at lunchtime and get some fresh air. Daylight and fresh air as such are incredibly invigorating and improve the appearance of your skin and make a big difference to your appearance as a whole.

# Conclusion: yes, it is possible to improve your acne

Suffering from acne is no fun – no matter if you are a teenager or an adult, female or male. Most of those who are affected feel insecure and ashamed of their acne, even though it is not their fault, and lack confidence when it comes to the opposite sex. But it is possible for them to regain at least some degree of control over their acne and get healthy skin again.

Even if your daily cleansing routine can sometimes be a pain and you could really do without visits at the dermatologist's – don't lose sight of your target. If you end up with beautiful pure skin and a look in the mirror proves that you finally have the kind of skin you always wanted, you will have to admit that it was worth the trouble.

And it is really not all that difficult. With a bit of practice reading labels is not complicated and becomes a habit after a while, and cleansing your skin and giving it additional moisture soon becomes everyday routine. If household remedies don't do the trick, your dermatologist can give you advice about the best medication and the most suitable treatment for your type of acne.

Many acne patients before you succeeded with one of the options described in this book and you too can have clear and healthy skin that you can be proud of. So what are you waiting for? Start today to care for your skin and treat it according to the methods described above. You too can be free of acne very soon.

Wishing you every success

Eva Beleco

**SECOND BOOK**

******

# The natural Approach
# to Beauty

Tips and recipes for natural beauty secrets -
how to keep your skin and body beautiful
and healthy without chemistry

******

# Introduction

Welcome to The Natural Approach to Beauty, a quick one-stop guide to achieving a life-transforming new you. Like many, you are most likely already tired of the temporary benefits that you are getting from the beauty products that you use, whether topical or taken orally. And that's not surprising.

Scarcely are cosmetics and other beauty products designed to make people look their best for the long haul. But what we all really want is skin that glows even without the BB Cream, skin that is naturally flawless and ready for flaunting whatever time of the day.

This book's aim is to bring you to a natural journey to achieve best skin that you can ever have, with tried and tested organic methods that have made a remarkable impact on the lives of many people, especially those that have been battling with skin problems for years.

If you are currently struggling with skin issues like rosacea, dermatitis, or—the most common of all—acne, this is the best skin restoration guide for you. This book is going to help you take control of your condition and get naturally beautiful skin for good.

You will know that you have successfully gone through this natural beauty approach because you

will notice significant changes in the overall appearance of your skin, not just on your face, but on your
whole body, as well as slowly manage to go out
without having to load your skin up with concealers
and other products to hide your blemishes.

At the same time, you should feel more rejuvenated, energized, and refreshed as you follow the
tips elaborated in this book and find it easier and
easier to maintain the kind of lifestyle that will keep
you looking the best possible you.

# Chapter 1:
# Hello Natural Beauty

So you have tried *everything* to make your skin look better, from topical treatments and creams to antibiotics. But nothing seems to work.

Our skin is highly individual. What product works for one person may not necessarily work for everyone. We have different skin types, and so it is very important to get to know our skin before trying any kind of treatment, especially if we are trying to control skin condition like severe acne or rosacea.

While most skin products today are accordingly labeled so that the people with the appropriate skin types only will use them, trying skin products out generally involves a trial and error process, where you will never know for sure what will work for you unless you try it. And when something doesn't work, the sad thing is that we often have to deal with our skin condition getting much worse than what it had been.

If you have been battling with severe skin problems for a long time, you know that this is not something that anyone will welcome, especially not you. We all want a cure.

What we want to achieve is natural beauty, the kind of skin that will no longer have to be aided by any chemically-formulated products that while they provide us some benefits actually possible harm us in some other ways.

The kind of treatments that we want to use are those that can provide lasting results without us having to experience any adverse side effects or threats to our health. This is where the natural, organic approach to beauty comes in.

For the purpose of discussion in this book, we define natural beauty as the pleasant and long-lasting overall condition of our skin and health without the use of chemicals and other chemically-formulated products.

Why is it so important that we opt for natural methods to achieve beautiful skin? Because while products may provide faster results, what they produce are scarcely long-lasting. Moreover, most products that people consider effective today can have adverse effects that make maintaining good skin tedious and, on some occasions, almost impossible.

Natural methods, on the other hand, while generally might take some time to produce significant results (not all), can provide results that will last and are easy to maintain. Natural methods also improve not only the condition of your skin but your health as a whole. Because they are natural, they do are safe to use and gentle on our skin. But aside from these great benefits, the use of organic methods and products also cost much less.

When we have long been exposed to beauty products and treatments that have such big price tags attached to them, cheap yet effective natural methods can be quite a breath of fresh air.

And because natural methods cost less, anybody anywhere can do them. Everyone should have access to ways to make their skin better. Our skin is the largest gland in our body, and it is the first and most noticeable thing that people see about us.

In the next chapter we are going to talk about why products and other chemical methods to achieving good skin is not the most ideal way to go about it.

Chapter 2:
# Why Organic Matters

Organic matters because it is safe and natural. Chemically formulated products merely try to encapsulate what natural products are already capable of doing. But the real issue is that these products contain ingredients that are potentially damaging to our health and may even worsen the very skin problems that we are trying to rid ourselves of.

Here is a list of chemical ingredients that are commonly found in different products that we use today, from shampoos to make-up, as well as powerful drugs that are used to clear the skin of blemishes and why we ought to steer clear from them.

## Sodium Laureth Sulfate (SLS)

Take the bottle of shampoo that you have in the bathroom, or the beauty soap that you use to cleanse your face. And then pay attention to the labels at the back where you can see the list of ingredients.

The next time you make a trip to the grocery store, try and take a look at the different products on the shelves and see what they are made of. You are most likely going to see this ingredient, sodium laureth sulfate or SLS, listed among the chemicals used to make the product.

SLS is a surfactant, which means that it relieves or eases the tension in between molecules. This is the reason why products like shampoos or cleansers create a lather when we apply them. This is what SLS does. And this is practically the reason why cosmetic companies have always incorporated SLS into the products that they manufacture. It makes products easier to apply.

SLS has so long been found used in various products, as a matter of fact, that we have come to associate a product's effectiveness in cleansing our hair or skin with how much lather it produces. The truth is, however, we do not really need the lather to cleanse. It only makes the cleansing process more enjoyable, yes, but it does not benefit us in the actual cleansing.

Now, SLS is also used in detergent soaps because of its capability to ease surface tension. For detergent products this is necessary because we are talking about removing deep-seated stains and cleaning out dirt from fabrics.

This kind of cleansing needs something tougher than what we would use to cleanse our skin. Before SLS was ever used for cosmetic products, it was used to make products that clean out vehicle tires and other machinery equipment, to remove stubborn grease, grime, and dirt that cling to the rubber.

Can you imagine an ingredient that is being used to clean rubber added into your daily facial cleanser? SLS is harsh on the skin and strips it of the natural oils that are meant to protect it from damage.

If you are currently suffering from moderate to extremely dry skin, you might want to try checking what your facial cleanser is made of. Although not yet scientifically proven to be a carcinogen, there are ongoing studies that claim that SLS can cause cancer when regularly made in contact with the skin.

So if SLS is this bad for the skin, you might be wondering why almost all cosmetics companies use this ingredient in their products. The answer is that SLS is a cheap ingredient that is easily accessible and can make products within reasonable rates for consumers. It makes products easy to create without having to incur too much cost.

## Parabens

There are a number of different kinds of paraben, such as methylparaben, propylparaben, and butylparaben. Paraben is a kind of preservative that is used to ensure long shelf life of cosmetic products.

To be fair, paraben is considered the better alternative in ensuring freshness of products; a while back, cosmetics companies used formaldehyde to preserve their products and "lock in" their effectiveness for as long as possible. Formaldehyde is the chemical that is used in embalming corpses and has long been found out unfit for skin beautification and maintenance.

However, there is an ongoing ruckus about whether or not parabens are also safe enough to be used for the skin, especially on a daily basis. If you have been paying attention to the products lined up at the department store, you would have noticed that there are a number of cosmetic lines that are now coming up with products that claim to be paraben-free.

If parabens were good enough, why would other lines even want to come up with products that are decidedly paraben-free, right? Because, to consider things fairly, parabens actually do a pretty good job in preserving especially the trickiest ones—lotions and creams.

One website, cosmeticsinfo.org, claims that certain kinds of parabens disrupt the normal function of the endocrine system and that when they come in contact with children, they can cause developmental dysfunctions and disorders.

The Food and Drug Administration of the United States have made several tests of parabens used in cosmetics and have come to the conclusion that parabens are relatively safe to use, which gave cosmetics companies the license to actually incorporate the preservative in their products. As much as 25 percent of paraben can be used in one product without causing any adverse side effects.

Long-term use of products with paraben, regardless of how much of the preservative it contains, however, might be a different issue altogether. The "Journal of Applied Toxicology" published in 2004 that parabens may have something to do with the development of breast cancer among women and interfering with the normal functions of the male reproductive system.

It has been found out that parabens actually copy the female hormone estrogen. This can be a problem because this can lead to the growth of estrogen-positive breast tumors, potentially leading to breast cancer.

The scientific discussion on how exactly parabens interact with our hormones is yet ongoing. And there are more studies to be conducted on the issue. However, the list of negative side effects that parabens can possibly cause should alert us to be more careful in our choice of products.

## Alcohol

Alcohol and its other forms can be found in many different skin products, such as toners, moisturizers, lotions, and cleansers. While not bad in itself, when applied to the skin, alcohol can be extremely drying.

People who have very oily skin might think that this is okay, that zero oil is the goal, and this is the ticket to get there. This, however, is wrong. Whether you have very oily skin or dry skin, you need oil or sebum.

People who have oily skin who try to dry out their skin too much are actually causing their oil glands to produce more sebum. The thing is that our skin needs a protective mantle of acidity and sebum in order to protect it from foreign particles, dirt, and other elements that can cause it damage. When we strip our skin completely of oil, our oil glands then work double hard to produce more oil. This is where the excess oiliness comes into the picture. This is the kind of oiliness that we do not want.

Those, on the other hand, who have naturally moderately dry to extremely dry skin will only make matters worse by applying products that contain alcohol. The excessive drying can lead to flaking and unsightly peeling. Very dry skin can also make wrinkles and fine lines appear more quickly and etch into the skin more deeply.

**Accutane or Roaccutane**

This powerful drug has been used by many people who have been plagued by severe acne for years. While it has been proven quite effective, there are extremely negative side effects that people who have used this drug can attest to, one of which is severe depression that leads to suicidal tendencies. There is a growing number of reports of people who have committed suicide after taking this drug.

Antibiotics, especially in large doses, are known to be very harsh on the body. So unless taken with the supervision of a doctor, they are to be avoided. Even dermatologists exercise great care in prescribing these drugs because of how potent they are, and only prescribe them when the cases is particularly severe. They are, therefore, a last resort.

While there has been a reported percentage of success from people who used either of these drugs, there are also quite a lot of people who do not see significant results from treating their condition using Accutane or Roaccutane.

Nothing, indeed, is a sure thing when it comes to treating skin problems as complicated to cure but as common as moderate to severe acne. So if you are not entirely sold out to using this drug, you might want to take a step back and consider a different route, because just like with taking any powerful drug regularly, taking Accutane or Roaccutane will eventually take a toll on your health as it tries to cure one skin problem.

**Perfume or Fragrance**

We all want products that smell good, but just like alcohol, the perfume added into the product can cause unnecessary drying. And also, the fragrance does not add to the effectiveness of the product, so it's not something that we really need.

People who have very sensitive skin may find that they react to certain products that contain fragrance. Just a little tip: If you are using a skin product, the less strong it smells, the gentler it is. So if you are looking for something that is not harsh, stay away from those that have fragrance in their list of ingredients.

Now that you have an idea about which ingredients to steer clear from, this is the time to go look into your beauty kit and check which products contain potentially harmful ingredients that might be doing your skin more harm than good.

To get started on your natural beauty journey, ditch these products and prepare to pamper yourself with 100 percent organic products that are safe to use and at the same time very effective.

# Chapter 3:
# Organic Beauty Product Alternatives

Excited to try out organic alternatives to those products that you have just thrown into the bin? There are plenty of different organic products that you can begin trying today, from products for face care, skin care, hair care, and even to aid in slimming down. Let's get started.

## Organic Facial Cleansers

Your face is the first thing that people see about you. And beautiful, glowing skin can greatly affect a person's self-esteem or confidence. With proper care, you can have skin as if you regularly had spa treatments, but without having to spend loads of money. These organic facial cleansers are not only cheap, they are most likely already present in your kitchen.

### Honey

Plain old natural honey is a true gem for skin care. It can work wonders because of its anti-inflammatory and anti-bacterial properties. If you have open wounds or cuts on your face, honey can hasten the healing process and quickly make it look like the cut was never there. People who have sensitive, acne-prone, or broken out skin will definitely find that honey is just short of a miracle product.

When buying honey to use as a facial wash, pick only that which is certified pure, raw, or organic. There are different kinds of honey to choose from, but the one that most people have had great success with is manuka honey. If you do not find this kind at your local supermarket or store, you can order it online.

It might sound strange to use a sweetener to cleanse your face, right? But given its wonderful properties, it has more to give than most facial cleansers that are out on the market.

And because it is very gentle, it will not cause any reaction, unless in the rare occasion that you are allergic to it.

**How to Use It:** Cleansing your face with honey is very simple. All you have to do is wet your face and squirt a few drops of honey onto your palm. If you keep your honey in the fridge it is bound to be a bit cool. Let it warm on your palm.

This should not take more than a few seconds. And then massage the honey all over your face in gentle circular strokes until you have covered every area of your face. To soak up its nourishing capabilities more, you can leave the honey on your face for three to five minutes before rinsing. Rinse your face with warm water and then pat dry.

Don't worry; honey easily comes off, so you should not be worried about whether you would be able to wash if off quickly. The honey facial wash makes your skin feel smooth and soft. In fact, you no longer need to moisturize after doing this method, because the honey is moisturizing enough on its own already. When done regularly, there should be a significant improvement in the texture of your skin and in skin conditions like acne.

## Oatmeal

Don't like to eat oatmeal? It's fine, just use it to wash your face. Oatmeal is another great organic cleanser that is very effective in improving the condition of the skin. You can use any kind of oatmeal that you can buy at the store. The instant ones are softer so they are generally preferably for facial cleansing.

Oatmeal works great because it has mild exfoliating and anti-inflammatory properties. It can easily shed the dry layer of the skin while soothing inflamed or irritated skin. People who are struggling with very sensitive skin due to conditions like dermatitis, rosacea, or severe acne can benefit a great deal from using oatmeal as a facial wash. It can reduce the skin's redness and calm it down. When you are having a breakout and you want to do something to make the inflammation go away faster, this should be a must-do.

**How to Use It:** To cleanse your face with oatmeal, take about a spoonful of oatmeal and clamp it in your wet fist, until the oatmeal turns into what looks like a mushy ball. And then, on your wet face, massage the oatmeal all over in a gentle circular motion.

Make sure not to press too hard, especially if you have active acne. Just massage very gently. The wet oatmeal should be soft to the skin. Afterwards, rinse your face thoroughly with warm water.

Because washing with oatmeal can be a bit messy, you might want to do this wearing an old shirt or when you are about to take a shower. Just like the honey, this is safe to do every day. With regular use, oatmeal can make the skin look brighter, suppler, and less inflamed.

## Oatmeal and Honey

If honey alone and oatmeal alone are wonderful to use as facial cleansers, using them together is even better. Using honey and oatmeal mixed together as an alternative to facial soap or facial wash is very rejuvenating for the skin and at the same time very soothing and calming.

This is a great alternative for those who are experiencing a new breakout, severely irritated skin, or skin suffering from an allergic reaction from using harsh chemicals or applying other products that contain allergens. The healing properties of honey combined with the calming effects of oatmeal work great to reduce irritation and itchiness, make swelling or inflammation go down, and lessen pain.

**How to Use It:** To make this organic facial cleanser, get a clean container, preferably a small bowl. Pour a small amount of oatmeal and add a few drops of honey. With your hands mix the two ingredients together by simply crushing the oatmeal with honey in your palm until the two have what looks like a soft oatmeal ball.

Wet your face and apply the honeyed oatmeal onto your face in gentle circular strokes, massaging the mixture in, making sure that you do not apply too much pressure. Afterwards, rinse your face thoroughly with warm water and then pat your skin dry.

When using this facial cleanser, you will want to keep your hair off your face with a headband. It can be a bit messy to use, but if you have the patience to add this cleansing method in your daily beauty regimen, you will surely not regret it after seeing the results.

**Plain Water**

If you stayed in the house the whole day and do not really need heavy duty cleansing, why not simply splash cool water on your face? Water alone is cleansing enough, plus it is definitely gentle on your skin. Do this only, however, when you did not apply any cream, make-up, or lotion.

Water alone can refresh your skin, but it is not capable of thoroughly removing products that you previously applied. To maximize its refreshing effects, make sure to wash your face with cool water.

## Organic Facial Scrubs

A good, gentle facial scrub is necessary to remove deep-seated dirt and dead skin cells as well as make sure that our skin looks bright and glowing. You can personally make your own facial scrubs at home without having to spend a lot of money on expensive beauty products.

Most, if not all, of the ingredients that you are going to use for the following scrubs are bound to be already found in your kitchen at home, and you can easily whip these up in minutes and use them right away.

It is advisable to make a fresh scrub each time so as to ensure the freshness of the scrub and make sure that you get all of the nourishing qualities from the organic ingredients that you are going to use. But for other scrubs, like the baking soda scrub, you don't even have to spend time for preparation. These are all easy, quick, and cheap but natural facial scrubs that you can make yourself at home.


**Baking Soda**

Even if you are not keen on baking, you still probably have this ingredient in your home. This versatile ingredient can be used for different purposes—baking, cleaning, whitening, and now even as a good facial scrub.

Baking soda is gentle and yet very effective at removing dirt that is trapped in the pores, making them look smaller after scrubbing, and exfoliating the skin to expose one that is healthy, soft, and smooth. What's great about this scrub is that it is very gentle on the skin, so you can even use it as your daily exfoliator, to be used once every day, to reveal brighter-looking skin.

**How to Use It:** Pour a tiny amount of baking soda in a small, clean bow. Add a few drops of water and mix them well with a clean spoon until you have a paste. Make sure that the consistency is just right. It should not be too runny or too dry. If the paste is too runny, add a little bit of baking soda. If it's too dry or thick, add one or two more drops of water.

When using this scrub, make sure that you have already cleansed your face. While your skin is still wet, apply the baking soda paste on your skin with your fingertips and massage it very gently. Be careful not to apply so much pressure or this will irritate your skin, especially if your skin is particularly sensitive.

Take note that while this is called a facial scrub, you don't really "scrub" your face with it, but instead massage it. Simply work the mixture on your skin in soft circular strokes until you have covered every area of your face. This scrub will effectively remove not just dead skin cells but even blackheads and other trapped dirt, such as any reside from make-up.

If you have breaks in the skin or lesions that are open and are yet fresh, it is not advisable to use this scrub, because it might only make the lesions worse.

But if you still want to use this scrub despite, you may do so by avoiding those areas of your skin that are open.

## Sea Salt

If you love going to the beach, you might have noticed that when you dip into the water while having a cut or a wound, it heals so much faster (although it can sting a mighty lot, mind you!). Sea salt is indeed a very effective antiseptic that can make the healing process so much faster.

If you are experiencing a breakout, this scrub can be very helpful in bringing the inflammation down and even close up those pimples that are open. It's great for those big, red cystic pimples that just won't go away too. Like baking soda, sea salt is also effective in removing deep-seated dirt from the skin's pores.

**How to Use It:** To use natural sea salt as a facial scrub, put a small amount in a clean container and add a few drops of water. Wash your face using a gentle cleanser—honey or oatmeal, perhaps?

Do not dry your skin. Get a clean container and put a small amount of sea salt into it. Add a few drops of water and then gently massage the sea salt in a circular motion on your skin using your fingertips.

If you have any open pimples it will sting a bit, just like when you dip into the sea with a wound on your leg. Don't worry, though; that sting is just like the one you experience when you apply medicine on a cut.

Be careful that you do not tear the already open skin by not apply much pressure, giving extra care on those open areas. Massage around the cut and simply let the salt work its way into the cut instead.

This is great to use if you want to speed up the healing process and shrink up any active pimples quickly. The sea salt can be quite drying, however, so remember not to use this facial scrub daily.

Use this scrub twice or thrice a week at most. If you have very oily skin the sea salt, though, can be helpful to bring the oiliness of your skin under control.

## Coffee Grounds

Need a caffeine boost every morning? Now, you don't have to throw out the coffee grounds that are left behind from a fresh brew. Just as a delicious cup of coffee can wake you up, you can use coffee grounds to wake your skin up.

For those times when you notice that you have puffy skin from lack of sleep or from being too tired, you can make your skin look like you have just been on a holiday. When applied on the skin, coffee also has slimming effects. It can enhance the contours of your face and make your face look tighter and slimmer. Don't be surprised if after using this scrub people will start asking you what product you have been using on your face.

**How to Use It:** Simply collect the left-behind coffee grounds from your latest brew and massage it on your freshly washed face with gentle circular strokes. If you want to use the coffee grounds that you are not able to use up for the next day, you can just put those away in a container and keep it in the fridge.

After scrubbing with the coffee grounds, rinse your face thoroughly with warm water and then pat your skin dry.

## Powdered Milk

If the bewitching Cleopatra was said to have bathed in milk, there has to be something about this dairy product that we need to get dibs of, don't you think? Milk naturally has lactic acid that can gently slough off dead skin cells and make the skin look softer and smoother.

This is a great scrub to use if you have dry, flaky skin. It can soothe irritated skin and relieve any redness as well. Using this scrub regularly can also improve the quality of your complexion and eventually give you what people call a milky translucent glow.

**How to Use It:** Powdered milk is very gentle and so it can be used whenever you want, as often as you want to. After washing your face with a gentle facial cleanser, you can use this scrub afterwards.

What you can do is pour a small amount of powdered milk, preferably the full cream kind (the fuller the milk is, the better it is for the skin), into a small bowl. To scrub, scoop some powdered milk with your fingers and massage it onto your skin in a circular motion.

When you have covered every area of your face, you can choose to either leave it on your face for a couple of minutes before washing or rinse right away.

The former option is a better option for those who want to relieve dry skin. To rinse thoroughly, use warm water, making sure there is nothing of the powdered milk left on your skin.

## Oatmeal

You just have to love oatmeal. It's not only nutritious, it has plenty of great uses to improve the quality of your skin. Aside from using oatmeal as a facial cleanser, you can also use it as a facial scrub. The ground oatmeal or the instant kind (any brand will do) is soft on the skin and so it can be used daily. As was earlier mentioned in this book, oatmeal is very effective because of its anti-inflammatory properties and its soothing effects.

**How to Use It:** To use oatmeal as a facial scrub, simply pour a little amount of oatmeal into a clean bowl (it should be a little less than a single helping). After washing your face thoroughly with a gentle cleanser, scoop some oatmeal with your fingers and massage it onto your face with circular strokes. Oatmeal is wonderful as an exfoliator and can instantly brighten the skin up as well. After you have thoroughly massaged the oatmeal on your face, rinse it off with warm water.

Warm water removes the oatmeal more quickly, so it makes things much easier, important especially if you want to speed things up if you don't have too much time to spare.

**Brown Sugar**

Have dry, flaky skin? When you look in the mirror and think that you look tired, you might need a little skin pick-me-upper. And brown sugar is the easy, effective, and inexpensive answer to that. Brown sugar can exfoliate the skin without being harsh.

Aside from tasting sweet, brown sugar can remove dead skin cells as well as clean out your pores from all the gunk that the week has dumped into them. This is also a very easy way to shrink your pores and give your skin a glow.

**How to Use It:** After cleansing your face, pour a small amount of brown sugar into a container and scoop out a tiny bit using your fingertips and massage the sugar into your skin in a gentle circular motion. Take your time in doing this, and be as gentle as possible while at the same time making sure that you allow your skin to be fully nourished by the scrub.

It can be a little sticky to apply, especially when you thoroughly massage it on your skin. So to wash it off, rinse with warm water, and then pat your skin dry. You will notice that your skin feels so much softer and smoother after using this scrub.

## Organic Hair Cleansing

To achieve that beautiful look, we should not pay attention to just our skin. Our hair, they say, is our crowning glory, and so it should be kept shiny and bouncy all the time.

That, however, has proven to be quite a challenge to a lot of people. Unless you were born with perfect hair, it will take quite an effort in order to keep your hair looking great. Fortunately, you don't have to spend so much money in order to achieve that salon-gorgeous hair.

This organic hair care regimen is effective and yet is very easy and cheap. Most of the products that you will be using are most likely already present in your kitchen. So here's how to get that perfect hair.

### Use Honey as an Organic Shampoo

We have already mentioned the amazing properties of this golden gem. What's more amazing is that we can use honey not only to make our skin look great. We can use it to cleanse our hair too. It can sound strange to those who have not tried it yet, but honey is truly a wonderful alternative to the chemical-loaded shampoos that we normally buy from the store.

You might be worried about the stickiness of the honey. You don't need to. When mixed with water, honey easily comes off and can be washed off from your hair quite easily.

In order to make shampooing with honey more convenient, put it in a squeezable container. Or better yet, buy a bottle that you are going to use solely as a shampoo and facial cleanser, so you can just keep it in the bathroom the whole time.

To use it, apply honey on thoroughly wet hair and massage onto your scalp. And then smooth the honey from the roots of your hair down to the tips until you have applied honey all over your hair. If you have plenty of time in your hands, you can leave the honey on for a while before washing it off. Rinse it off thoroughly and then squeeze the water off your hair to prepare for the next step.

**Condition with Apple Cider Vinegar**

Apple cider vinegar is practically the rave (next to honey) among organic product enthusiasts. It has so many health benefits and has plenty of advantages when incorporated into your beauty regimen. But let's not get ahead of ourselves and focus on how we can make our hair look great with this amazing product.

Our ordinary conditioners claim that they can make our hair look shiny and smooth and soft. But while they can actually do that, there are several downsides that actually outweigh the benefits that they are able to provide.

Many people experience too much hair fall, thinning of the hair, and other negative effects from using store bought conditioners on a regular basis. The good news is that apple cider vinegar can produce the results that we wish to get with ordinary conditioners and even better.

ACV can make the hair look shiny and very soft to the touch. After using it and seeing the results, you will start wondering why not everybody is using it as a conditioner instead of those cheap conditioners that people buy at the grocery store.

To condition with apple cider vinegar, simply mix one part apple cider vinegar and one part water in a ready container. Mix the two and then pour it onto your scalp and hair that had just been washed with honey. To maximize the benefits of apple cider vinegar, leave it on for a few minutes, keeping your hair kept inside a shower cap. Afterwards, rinse the apple cider off thoroughly.

At this point you might be concerned about the smell. Apple cider vinegar, just like any kind of vinegar, has a pretty strong smell, but don't you worry; the smell goes away pretty fast. By the time your hair had dried, you will notice that there is no longer any smell.

And the best part is that when you touch your hair, you will be absolutely amazed by the softness of your hair and how shiny it looks. The effects are way better than when you used ordinary conditioner.

In order to keep your hair in the best condition, try to wash your hair every other day rather than every day. When we wash our hair that often it has the natural tendency to dry out, and what we should want is to keep it with just the right amount of natural oil so that it looks shiny and soft.

If your hair is not particularly oily, you can even shampoo instead every two days. It all depends on how your hair responds. Try to observe which one your hair responds better to and stick to that.

Also, as your hair is trying to get used to the new routine, especially that of the use of honey as a shampoo, make some allowances to the fact that it feels different from using ordinary products. Also, the process of using these organic products can take a bit of getting used to, so allow yourself some time to adjust to the new process of washing your hair. Your hair will definitely thank you for sticking to the routine.

## Organic Toners

Toners are necessary in order to keep your skin tone even. When we experience skin issues like breakouts, the inflammation that they bring can produce the skin tone to become uneven.

There are parts that might look redder than others, and acne or rosacea can leave marks that can be either red, purple, or brown. All of these are very unsightly. Organic toners can help to balance out the skin tone and fade marks and lighten scars.

### Apple Cider Vinegar

This amazing ingredient is capable of evening out your skin tone with consistent use. It is important, however, to pick only raw, organic apple cider vinegar to use as your toner, and not the kind that we use to prepare salads and cook dishes.

The most highly recommended brand of apple cider vinegar is Bragg's, because it has the "mother" in it, which is what gives it its murky brown appearance. The "mother" in the apple cider vinegar contains most of the nutritious content that will aid in making sure the ACV is effective for the skin.

**How to Use It:** Just like any kind of vinegar, ACV is highly acidic and should be used the right way in order for it to not burn the skin or cause any unwanted effects. To create your own apple cider vinegar toner, get a clean unused bottle and pour one part ACV and eight parts distilled water.

This ratio is good as a starter, to help your skin get used to the toner. You would not want to use a high concentration right away as it might produce bad results instead of good ones. You can use this first bottle of toner for the first week of use, and then slowly increase the concentration of the toner to the ratio that you think your skin responds to best. It is essential to increase the amount of apple cider vinegar slowly, so that you are sure that your skin is ready.

Using a cotton ball, apply the toner gently in upward strokes. With consistent use, you should see a significant improvement in your complexion and in the overall tone of your skin. Any blemish marks such as scars and pimple marks should also become lighter and lighter from using this toner.

**Green Tea**

Green tea is a powerful antioxidant that is widely talked about because of the good benefits that we can get from drinking it regularly. Aside from drinking a cup of green tea every day, however, you can also use it as a gentle natural toner. If you don't want to take your chances with the apple cider vinegar, or if you simply can't tolerate its smell, this is the perfect alternative.

It is very gentle on the skin, and it nourishes without the danger of being too harsh, even when prepared in high concentrations.

**How to Use It:** To use green tea as a toner, boil some water. Put a bag of green tea in a mug and then pour water into it. You would not want to pour too much water.

As a matter of fact, the lesser the amount of water, the better it is. It becomes more effective in high concentrations, and you would want to soak up as much nourishment from the green tea as possible.

Leave it to brew for a few minutes and let it cool. Once it is a tolerable temperature, pour it into a clean bottle. Put a few drops of this toner onto a cotton ball and apply it onto your skin in gentle upward strokes.

Keep the bottle in the fridge to keep it fresh. But in order to make sure that you always have a fresh toner available, replace the toner with a fresh brew every week.


## Sea Salt

Sea salt has amazing healing properties. So this toner is particularly effective for those who have lesions on their face, any allergy, irritated or burned skin from using harsh chemicals, or any kind of cut.

It will sting for a few minutes, but don't worry about it. It's just the sea salt working its magic and restoring your skin. This toner, however, has the tendency to draw moisture from the skin, so it is great for those who have cystic acne that they want to dry out, and it should be prepared in just right concentration so as not to make other parts of the face too dry.

**How to Use It:** To prepare this toner, get a clean unused bottle and fill it up to a third with distilled water. Afterwards, pour sea salt just enough to cover the entire bottom of the bottle. You would not want the mixture to be too highly concentrated or it will make your skin very dry. Mix it up until the salts are completely dissolved in the water.

Use a cotton ball to apply it onto your face in gentle upward strokes. You can use this toner twice a day, once in the morning after cleansing, and once at night before bedtime. You should have no problem with applying any make-up on top of this toner.


## Organic Body moisturizers

If your face deserves meticulous care, skin on the rest of your body does too. Thankfully, skin on our body is generally not as sensitive as skin on our face, and so we don't have to take the same rigorous cleansing methods that we take to wash our face and keep it looking its best.

The trick, however, for the rest of our body is that of keeping it moisturized right. It is absolutely possible to have skin that is firm, soft, and glowing, without having to go to the spa.

You can do wonders for your skin right inside the comfort of your own home, and the things that you can use are all natural, effective, and again, amazingly inexpensive, as compared to most beauty products. The following are the best skin moisturizers that you can use on a daily basis, even twice a day.


**Coconut Oil**

Coconut oil is a wonder ingredient. It can practically work miracles especially for those who are plagued with excessively dry, flaky, or irritated skin. When you want to nourish your skin and keep it moisturized, this is a good natural product to use instead of the products that you can buy at Body Shop or from any skin care line.

**How to Use It:** It is very easy to use. After a bath, just massage a tiny amount of coconut oil all over your body. Make sure not to use too much coconut oil, especially if you are applying it in the morning, if you don't want to look too shiny.

A few drops of coconut oil can go a long way, so just about that amount will do for the whole body. At night, however, you can lather as much coconut oil as you want on your skin, because you're going to bed anyway, and you shouldn't be bothered about it making your skin look too shiny or it feeling too thick on your skin.

To soften parts of your skin that are particularly tougher, such as the soles of the feet, you can lather a liberal amount of coconut oil on this particular area and cover your feet up with a good pair of thick cotton socks. When you wake up in the morning, you will notice a significant improvement in the softness of your skin.

### Extra Virgin Olive Oil

Olive oil is another product that many women use for beautification. It has great moisturizing properties because it locks in the moisture of the skin to make it look supple and keep the complexion looking beautiful.

Compared to coconut oil, extra virgin olive oil can cost a bit more, but the effects that you get from this wonderful product make the cost definitely worth it. It is a very light ingredient, so if you prefer that kind of consistency rather than a thick one, it's perfect for you.

Like when applying coconut oil, you can use only a few drops of extra virgin olive oil for all over your body. Because it is light, it's wonderful to use particularly at daytime, when you are going out. It doesn't make the skin look too oily, but it keeps it looking supple and just a little shiny that you don't have to use any other lotion to make you look gorgeous.

## Organic Facial Moisturizers

Even if you have oily skin, you should not skip this essential step. What a lot of people make the mistake of doing is that when they think they have oily skin, they refuse to moisturize, thinking that it will only make their skin too oily.

When we dry out your skin, our oil glands work twice as hard to produce the necessary sebum in order to create a protective mantle on the skin that will keep damaging elements at bay. Moreover, our skin needs the proper moisture in order to keep it supple and soft.

It is very important to take note that most of the time, what makes the skin easily irritated is that it is too lacking in moisture. These organic moisturizers can help you lock in moisture in your facial skin. This also wards away those fine lines and wrinkles that most women dread.

## Extra Virgin Olive Oil

This great product is great to use not only for the body. It is gentle enough to be applied regularly on the face, and because of its very light texture, you can apply this in the morning and put on make-up over it just as if you were using an ordinary facial moisturizer. But unlike ordinary facial moisturizers, this does not contain any potentially harmful chemicals.

**How to Use It:** After applying your organic toner and letting it dry, get a drop or two of extra virgin olive oil and massage it onto your face. It is important to work it all over your face gently in small circular strokes.

You can apply this also around the eye area to take control of wrinkles and fine lines. However, take caution when doing so, because the skin around the eyes is very sensitive. Avoid stretching at the skin around this area. Instead, pat the olive oil on.

You will know that you applied too much because your skin will look too shiny and it will be hard to put make-up on top of it. The ideal amount is just a tiny drop or two. This should just create a smooth film on your skin, and should not make your face look too oily.

If you are suffering from acne or other skin problems, extra virgin olive oil can soothe the inflammation and even fade acne scars and even your skin tone. You can see better results when you use this facial moisturizer every day.

**Adding Tea Tree Oil**

There are those pesky times when we look in the mirror and find that we have a breakout. Nobody wants a breakout. But somehow, they keep bothering many of us. If you find that there are a few pimples just about to surface on your skin, you can keep them from fully showing up by adding tea tree oil into your organic facial moisturizer.

Tea tree oil is a wonderful anti-bacterial and anti-inflammatory that can keep acne at bay. The best time to take control of acne is when it is just about to pay you a visit. To make your own olive oil and tea tree oil facial moisturizer, just prepare a small clean bottle.

Pour in the olive oil up to the third of the bottle. Add a few drops of the tea tree oil. The amount of tea tree oil that you add will depend on the size of the bottle or how much olive oil you use. Tea tree oil is pretty effective even in small amounts, so you would not want to waste it by putting too much.

**How to Use It:** To use this mixture, apply just as you would plain extra virgin olive oil.

## Coconut Oil for Nighttime Moisturizing

The texture of coconut oil is quite thicker than that of olive oil, but coconut oil is a great moisturizer, with amazing healing properties as well.

So if you want the benefits of coconut oil but not the thickness, which is not very convenient for daytime use, you can use it at night, right before you go to bed. Coconut oil is extra hydrating and is an excellent alternative to night creams.

**How to Use It:** Apply a liberal amount of coconut oil on your face after cleansing it thoroughly and

patting it dry. Leave it on overnight to get the maximum benefits. Wash it off in the morning with warm
water. You can see for yourself how soft your skin
becomes after this nighttime moisturizing.

# Chapter 4:
# Battling Common Skin Issues

No matter how well we take care our skin, there will always be times when we are going to battle through skin problems. If you have been struggling with a skin problem for a long time, you are probably desperate to find a cure.

Although organic skin treatments will not produce instant results, they will definitely provide significant improvement and consistently improve the condition of your skin with regular use. Also, unlike with prescription medication and other harsh chemicals that are used to treat skin issues, these organic treatments will nourish your skin and keep further ski problems at bay.

## Acne, Rosacea, Allergic Reactions, Excessive Dryness

The most common skin issue is acne. Acne is characterized by pimple breakouts that leave dark acne marks and scars. Acne can be caused by various things, such as genes, diet, poor health, sleep deprivation, stress, and hormonal imbalance.

When treating acne, it is very important to get to the root of the problem. In order to come up with an effective cure, you have to know exactly what it is that's causing the acne breakout, especially if it is recurring and has been there for quite a while now.

However, certain topical treatments can improve the condition of the skin and make the pimples go away faster and make the scars fade more quickly. These treatments are also helpful in treating skin problems like acne, rosacea, allergic reactions, and dryness.

## Oatmeal and Honey Face Mask

We are already acquainted with the effectiveness of honey and oatmeal individually as well as together.

A combination of these power ingredients can cystic pimples shrink in size as well as calm inflamed skin. Together, the honey and oatmeal can also reduce the redness of the skin and shrink cystic pimples.

**How to Use It:** Cook the oatmeal just as you would if you were going to eat it. If you are using instant oatmeal, the easier and quicker it will be for you to prepare. Stir it until it becomes pasty in consistency and then add a few drops of honey.

While it is still warm—take not: not hot—apply it all over your face. Be as generous as you can be in the application. The thicker the coverage, the better it is, especially if you are dealing with severe acne with cystic pimples. Leave this mask on until it becomes stiff and dry. You will know that it is thoroughly dry because it will become crusty.

When it does, wash it off with warm water, massaging the mixture on your face gently so as to maximize the benefits of the mask. Make sure that there is no residue of the mask left on your skin. And then pat your face dry.

## Honey Face Mask

Honey works wonders by itself. And if you have any open and active pimples on your face, this if the perfect product to help it close up and heal faster. The anti-inflammatory properties of honey make it very useful for different kinds of skin ailments.

**How to Use It:** After cleansing your face and patting it dry, massage your face with honey in gentle circular strokes. Leave this coating of honey on for as long as you like. If you have nothing to do for the day and can afford to stay home, you can leave it on your skin the whole day and even overnight. The longer it stays on your skin, the better, because the more of its healing properties your skin gets to soak up.

If you intend to leave the mask on overnight, use a paper mask to cover it up and keep it from messing your pillows and sheets up. In the morning, rinse it off your skin thoroughly with warm water.

## Cocoa, Coffee, and Honey Face Mask

You would think this combination is only good for drinking. Well, it might be good for drinking too, but this delightful combo is definitely not just for your taste buds. Cocoa is rich in antioxidants that get rid of unwanted toxins from the skin, cleanses, and rejuvenates it.

Coffee, on the other hand is wonderful for waking the skin up and reviving it when it looks puffy and tired. These three, when mixed together and applied onto your face can make leave it feeling at refreshed, soft, and smooth.

**How to Use It:** To prepare this face mask, simply mix these three ingredients together. Mix one tablespoon of cocoa powder, one tablespoon of coffee or coffee grounds, a teaspoon of honey, and about a tablespoon of water in a clean bowl.

The consistency should be just like a paste. It should be thick so that it does not drip when you apply it on your face. You can leave it on for 20 to 30 minutes or until it becomes stiff and it becomes hard to move the muscles on your face. And then rinse it off thoroughly with warm water. You can do this face mask as often as you want for a more rejuvenated skin.

## Baking Soda Pimple Spot Treatment

Now back to baking soda. Another one of the ways by which you can use baking soda is as a simple yet effective spot treatment for any existing active pimples.

This is very effective to dry those pimples out and prevent them from becoming very red and enlarged. When doing this treatment, apply the baking soda strictly only on the pimples, because it will dry out your skin if you apply it elsewhere.

**How to Use It:** To prepare this spot treatment, mix a small amount of baking soda and a few drops of water in a clean bowl. Mix these thoroughly until you make a thick paste. It is important to make the consistency thick enough so that it does not slide off your face when you apply it.

When the mixture is ready, take a Q-tip and use it to apply the baking soda paste directly onto the blemishes. If the pimples are active and very red, they might sting a bit. But this stinging should go away in a few minutes. If the stinging does not go away and is not tolerable, wash it off right away. You might be allergic to baking soda, and it will only burn your skin.

**Sea Salt Pimple Spot Treatment**

For those pesky cystic pimples that have been sitting on your face for a while now and just refuse to go away, you can shoo them with this spot treatment. Sea salt can dry the pimple out and reduce its size significantly even after just one application.

This is one of the spot treatments that provide the fastest results. To consistently shrink the pimples, do this spot treatment every day and leave as long as possible during the day when you have the time to do so.

**How to Use It:** In a clean container, pour a small amount of natural sea salt and add a few drops of water. Make sure that the water is not too much to make the salt dissolve completely. The purpose of the water is just to aid the skin absorb the salt more easily as well as to let it stick to the skin more effectively.

To apply this on your skin, use a Q-tip and apply the sea salt crystals directly on the pimples. What this should look like is a tiny lump of salt on a pimple.

If you're wondering whether this will stick; the answer is yes, and so you don't have to worry about moving around, because as long as it was mixed with water, it will stay on your skin.

It is normal to feel a slight tingling sensation or even stinging on the areas where you applied the sea salt. But this stinging should be very tolerable and nowhere near painful. However, if you are applying it on an open pimple (which is okay, by the way, because the salt will simply close that pimple up and make it heal faster), it can sting a bit more.

Just let it be and leave it on for as long as you can. Soon enough, there should be no more of the tingling sensation left. For better results, you can leave the spot treatment on overnight and wash it off in the morning when you cleanse your face.


**Honey and Cinnamon Face Mask**

Worried about existing acne as well as the dark marks that previous breakouts left on your skin? This face mask should take care of that problem.

We are already familiar with honey. Cinnamon, on the other hand, is a very common ingredient that we use in our coffee, add to our bread recipes, and use for cooking. But aside from being a tasty ingredient, cinnamon has high anti-inflammatory as well as lightening properties that can fade your acne scars while it deals with the active ones.

It can prevent present breakouts from leaving nasty scars or dark marks on your face. Plus, together with honey, this smells just heavenly. And it tastes good too.

**How to Use It:** To prepare this mask, simply mix one tablespoon of cinnamon powder and one teaspoon of honey in a clean bowl. Carefully mix these ingredients thoroughly until you make a thick paste. You will notice that it can be a bit tricky to mix these two especially if the honey is not a lot. But keep carefully mixing until you get the right consistency.

To apply, you can use your fingertips or you can use an old but cleaned make-up brush. Apply it on your skin, covering every area of your face with a liberal amount of the mixture, leaving out only the eye areas. Leave this face mask for as long as you possible can let it.

The longer it stays on your skin, the better the results. So if you don't have to hang out with friends at night or leave the house, just keep it on. When it has stiffened, rinse it off thoroughly with warm water. If you prefer to leave it on overnight, rinse it off with warm water in the morning.

Use a paper mask over it, though, if you want to leave it on overnight, because it will stain your sheets.

**Honey, Cinnamon, and Turmeric Face Mask**

To take control of acne and at the same time hasten the process of lightening your acne scars, and other dark spots, you can use this effective facial mask.

Turmeric is a well-known spice used for various dishes but is also well touted in Ayurvedic medicine and has great lightening properties. It can make the skin instantly brighter and the scars to fade significantly with consistent use.

**How to Use It:** To prepare this face mask, mix one tablespoon of cinnamon powder, one teaspoon of turmeric powder, and about a tablespoon of honey in a clean bowl or container. Mix these ingredients well until you are able to reach a thick consistency. It should be stick enough to stay on your face when you apply it, and the ingredients should be properly mixed together.

To apply, you can use your fingers or an old but clean make-up brush, put a liberal amount of the mixture all over your face, excepting the general eye area. Take care not to apply the mixture on your eyebrows, because turmeric powder is also commonly used to remove or thin our hairs.

When the face mask becomes stiff on your face, or when it starts to crack, you can rinse it off thoroughly using warm water. You will notice that the face mask can leave a slight yellowish tinge on your skin.

This, however, goes away. But because of this, make sure that you do not apply this mask immediately before an appointment. You will need to have removed it already the night before if you have to go out during the day. Also, because the turmeric can stain, retrain from leaving it on overnight, or you will ruin both your sheets and your clothes.

If you want to lessen the staining quality of this mask, though, you can lessen the proportion of the turmeric that you add into the mixture. Or you can simply leave it on for a shorter period of time.

**Egg White and Lemon Juice Face Mask**

Egg white is an excellent ingredient for a face mask because it instantly gives the skin a small but instant face lift. It makes the skin tighter, smoother, and brighter. And lemon juice, of course, has the acidity to make it a good scar fading ingredient. This face mask is perfect for those who want to fade any blemishes or scars that are left behind from a breakout.

When combined, these two ingredients can help restore your skin's natural glow.

**How to Use It:** To make this face mask, make a small hole at one end of an egg and let the egg white out, careful not to let the egg yolk come out as well. Whisk the egg white until it foams. Slice a lemon in half and squeeze the juice of one half into the whisked egg white. Mix these two thoroughly.

Using an old but clean make-up brush, apply the mixture onto your whole face, except the eye area. Let this face mask to dry on your skin. You will know that it has dried because it will stiffen on your face. Once this happens, rinse the mask off with warm water. Be careful not to leave any residue of the face mask on your skin. Pat dry.

If you don't want the egg yolk to go to waste, you can also use it right after you have washed the egg white mask off. Simply whisk the egg yolk and using a clean make-up brush apply it onto your face, leaving it until dries. This face mask will moisturize your skin. Egg yolk has excellent moisturizing properties, so it is a nice follow-up to the egg-white and lemon mask.

**Milk Powder and Lemon Juice Face Mask**

To nourish your skin and at the same time deal with the dark spots on your skin, use full cream milk powder and lemon as a face mask. Milk has lactic acid which is capable of gently exfoliating the skin and removing dead skin cells.

While it exfoliates the skin, it is also capable of nourishing it and locking in moisture. Lemon juice is perfect to fade those stubborn pimple marks and other dark spots.

**How to Use it:** Take one two tablespoons of milk powder (or more if you want) and about a teaspoon of lemon juice. Mix the two ingredients together and add a few drops of water, just enough to make the consistency to the mask thick enough to make it stick to your skin. When the mask is ready, you can apply it on your face using your fingers or an old cleaned make-up brush. Leave the mask on until it has dried. And then wash it off with warm water.

**Yogurt or Sour Milk Face Mask**

Is there any left behind milk that has gone bad in your kitchen? Don't throw that away! You can use sour or slightly spoiled milk for your skin. That is an excellent source of lactic acid, even better than milk that is still good for drinking. Aren't you glad that there finally is something for which you can put that spoiled milk to good use?

**How to Use It:** To use sour milk as a face mask, wash your face with a gentle cleanser. After patting your skin dry, apply this face mask using your fingertips or a make-up brush. Leave it on until it has dried. But if you want to, you can also leave it on overnight.

Milk, when it has dried, becomes this light film on your skin and is not particularly bothersome. But to be sure that you do not mess the sheets, you can put a paper mask over it. In the morning, wash it off using warm water or wash as usual.

Many people can attest to the wonderful skin nourishing properties of sour milk. And when you do this mask consistently, it will significantly improve your complexion, even out your skin tone, fade blemishes and acne marks, and even keep pimples at bay. Wonderful, isn't it?

## Lemon Juice Spot Treatment

To hasten the fading of those pimple marks and blemishes, you can do a lemon juice spot treatment. However, because of the high level of acidity of lemon juice, you should not leave this on overnight. The maximum time you should leave it on is 20 minutes.

Acid can irritate the skin when made in contact with the skin in high concentrations. But when done properly, lemon juice can sure lighten those dark spots until you can barely tell that they were ever there.

**How to Use It:** This spot treatment is mostly for dark spots and scars, but you can also apply this to active pimples in order to dry them out and help them heal and shrink faster. To use, simply squeeze the juice out of a fresh lemon into a clean container.

Get a Q-tip and dip it into the lemon juice. Use this to apply the lemon juice on any of the areas that you want to fade or dry up. Leave it on for 15 to 20 minutes and then wash it off with water.

You can repeat this process twice a day every day, once in the morning and once at night before you go to bed.

## Garlic Spot Treatment

This spot treatment is great for cystic pimples and pimples that are yet about to surface. Garlic has strong anti-bacterial properties, and when it is crushes or sliced, it produces a substance called allicin that has stronger antioxidant properties than green tea. When used to spot treat pimples, they will easily dry up

**How to Use It:** To use garlic, get one fresh clove of garlic and peel it. Slice a thin layer off one end of the clove and then pat this fleshy part directly on the pimple. The trick is not to let it stay on top of the pimple. Garlic can easily burn sensitive skin, so leaving it on the skin is not a very good idea.

Also, do not rub it on the pimple, or you will tear the skin and cause it to leave the mark. Just pat it on the pimple a few times. You will notice that you feel a slight stinging sensation while doing this. Keep patting the garlic on the pimple for a minute. Do not wash your face after this. It is preferable that you had already washed and cleansed your face before spot treating your pimples with garlic.

Garlic has a pretty strong smell, so if you can't stand it, you can splash some water on your face after the spot treatment. But don't use soap. Just splash some water on your face until the smell goes away or becomes tolerable.

# Chapter 5:
# Skin Habits to Do Without

Now that we have exhaustively talked about how you can pamper your skin, this is the time to discuss certain skin habits that most people have that we should get rid of. If you notice that you yourself have these habits, you can now actively do something to keep yourself from doing them again.

## Picking at Newly Healed Pimples

The nature of the skin's healing process is just that right after a wound has closed up, there will appear a darker colored scan on the area that has just healed.

The tendency for most of us is to pick at this newly healed pimples, exposing the part underneath that is just on the process of being restored. What happens when we pick at them is we cause the wound to open up again and trigger more pigmentation that naturally occurs when trauma on the skin has occurred.

We don't want to have to deal with any scars. But when we pick at pimples, both active and newly healed is that we increase the probability of hyperpigmentation and scarring. When the scarring becomes indented, there is little that can be done to restore it to how it used to look like, so it is definitely much better to leave the skin alone and let it restore itself in peace.

**Tolerating Sleep Deprivation**

Sleep is a very important beauty element. No matter how many products you load up on your skin, as long as you are not allowing your body to naturally recuperate and rejuvenate, you will look stressed and increase the chances of having a breakout. If you are acne-prone, sleep should be your best friend. If you have a busy schedule, try your best to squeeze in a good eight hours of sleep every day, if you want to take your acne under control.

We have to understand that what is happening on the surface is largely because of what is happening on the inside. If your body is stressed, it will naturally react like a stressed body reacts. And because fatigue causes the body's immunity to become low, you are exposing yourself to every chance there is to worsen the condition of your skin.

## Using Different Products at the Same Time

Do not confuse your skin. Help it recover by sticking to a specific skin regimen that you have observed works well for you. The problem with using many different products at the same time or changing from one product to another too often, especially if you are using products that have harsh ingredients, is that you are not giving your skin the time to adjust to the product yet. Our skin is a lot like us. It needs time to get used to things that we introduce to it. So make allowances for that, and the moment you notice that something is working, stick to it.

Of course, using harsh chemicals on your skin is not doing it any good. The golden rule when it comes to skin is this: Be good to it and it will be good to you. Be gentle as you can be on your skin, and use only those products that you know will do the same.

## Applying Make-Up without Cleansing First

This is an absolute no-no. Make-up has the tendency to clog the pores, and when you do not cleanse before applying make-up, you trap the dirt and oil in your pores. Also cleansing your face before applying make-up will keep your brushes and other things clean, so that when you use them you do not irritate your skin with dirty tools.

In relation to this, keep your make-up brushes, powder puffs, and other personal things to yourself and do not let other people use them. You should take extra care to keep them hygienic, and if somebody needs a brush, you will just have to say that she has to buy her own, or else you might expect a breakout soon after, if your skin is sensitive.

**Sleeping with Make-Up On**

Just like applying make-up without washing your face, this should be something that no one ever does. When you sleep with make-up on, you allow the dirt from the whole day plus the make-up sit on your skin and mix with the natural sebum that your skin produces. This becomes something that can clog the pores and cause the skin to become extremely oily, trapping more dirt.

Be strict with your hygiene and make it a point that when you get home, you take all of your make-up off. This is very important especially for those who apply make-up on a daily basis. Cleansing your face right after gives your skin the chance to breathe.

**Not Replacing the Sheets Regularly**

If you want to keep your skin cleansed by bedtime, you will also want to have clean sheets to sleep on. People who are acne-prone or have very sensitive skin should make it a point to replace sheets every week in order to make sure that the oils that are collected on the sheets and other dust and dirt are gotten rid of. You would definitely not want to sleep on sheets that might cause you to break out in a fresh batch pimples pretty soon.

If replacing the sheets every week is a very tedious task to you, then at least replace the rest of the bed sheets twice a month, and replace only the pillow cases weekly. What's most important is that the sheets that get in contact with your face are clean.

If you notice that you have been breaking out a lot, you might also want to check whether you are allergic to the fabric in your sheets and consider buying hypo-allergenic ones. Aside from keeping acne at bay with keeping fresh sheets, you'll definitely sleep better with clean sheets on your bed.

## Not Drinking Enough Water

Water is the best toxin remover. And our bodies need to be properly hydrated in order to function properly. If you hardly drink any water throughout the day, you are seriously depriving your body something that it badly needs.

The ideal is to drink three to four liters of water a day. That can sound a lot, but when you make it a habit to drink water every now and then, you will find it becomes easier to do. One easy thing that will help you is to simply obey your thirst. Our bodies are like these intelligent machines. And when we feel thirsty, it is basically because we need to get more hydration.

Drinking plenty of water can affect the overall health of your organs, skin, and hair. Also, you will feel more energized by drinking more water.

# Chapter 6:
# Going Beyond Skin-Deep

It is necessary to always remember that whatever we do with the inside will eventually show on the outside. And so, no matter how well we take care of our skin on the surface, if we neglect what's beneath that, we're never going to get the lasting results that we want. We can't just take care of what's inside us and forget about taking care of our skin on the outside either. Both methods have to go hand in hand.

## Change Your Lifestyle for the Better

What beauty both on the inside and outside requires a lifestyle change. This guide is about making use of organic products for daily skin care and treatment, and so if you want to subscribe to this method, it will require you to turn back from the chemically formulated products that used to be in your beauty routine.

But equally important is a change in lifestyle. The kind of food that you feed yourself will tell on the condition of your skin. There are even famous and beautiful celebrities who can attest to the negative effects of not choosing what you eat. Cameron Diaz, for example, has become quite vocal about her struggles with acne as a young adult. She confessed to her bad eating habits, feeding herself fries, Big Macs and sodas almost all the time. She admitted to having terrible broken out skin as a result.

And what finally got her out of that was a total diet change. Now, she chooses what she eats and makes sure that she is nourishing her body on the inside aside from taking care of her body on the outside.

If celebrities who have all the resources at their disposal can still be plagued by skin conditions like moderate to severe acne when they do not pay attention to their health well enough, don't you think we also should pay more attention to our health?

This involves committing to regular exercise on top of eating the right kind of food. Treat your body well, and it will be good to you. You will thank yourself later for embarking on a positive lifestyle change, because of the amazing positive results that you will eventually reap.

## Limit Stressors

Another thing that we have to do in order to reap lasting positive results is to limit the stressors in our lives. Stress, although not proven scientifically to cause acne and other skin problems, most of us can attest to the fact that when we are stressed, we are more prone to get sick and breakouts.

If you are suffering from severe acne today and this is causing you a great deal of distress, first of all, you have to remember that the condition of your skin does not define you. You are beautiful. And you have to first believe that there is hope for you.

Many studies have found that acne and depression actually feed each other. The more you have acne, the more depressed you become, and the more depressed you become, the more you have acne. They practically trigger each other.

The only way to curb this phenomenon is to start living despite what you think is a good reason to keep you from living the kind of life that you want, meeting new people, experiencing exciting things. Determine to do things that you love and not be hindered by a temporary skin condition. Because, after all, it is temporary.

Things are going to get better. So get your face out of that paper bag and get out into the world. There are new, exciting things that await you.

Another thing that you can do to limit stressors is to determine to avoid situations that you know will not bring encouragement or that do not give you a sense of fulfilment and purpose. Hang out more with positive people who always see the brighter side of things.

**Drinking Apple Cider Vinegar**

This powerhouse can become a great health drink that can help in making sure we have clean guts and that can correct hormonal imbalance. For those who suffer from recurring acne due to hormonal imbalance, this is something that you might want to do on top of the topical skin treatments that you think are best for you.

For the purpose of this concoction, use only apple cider vinegar that is pure, organic, and natural. One of the best brands to use is Bragg's, because this one has the "mother" in the bottle and can give maximum health benefits compared to other brands of apple cider vinegar.

**How to Use It:** To prepare, get a 500 mL water bottle and fill it with distilled water. Afterwards, pour two capfuls of apple cider vinegar into the bottle. Shake the bottle until the apple cider is completely mixed with the water. You can drink this every day, once in the morning upon waking up, once before you go to sleep, and thirty minutes before every meal. If this becomes a bit tedious for you to remember to do, you can simply drink your apple cider vinegar in the morning and at night.

This not only corrects hormonal imbalance but also improves and speeds up metabolism, which means that every time you eat your food quickly gets converted into energy. This can helps a great deal when you are looking to slim down. Aside from that, you can also notice an improvement in your bowel improvement. Your stomach should feel lighter and cleaner.

## Drink Green Tea Daily

Green tea is a wonderful antioxidant that not only removes toxins from your system but also improves your metabolism and gives you more energy. If you have a demanding schedule all the time and you feel like you don't have as much energy as you need, you can make it a habit to drink two or more cups of green tea every day.

For those who are not much of tea drinkers, you might find green tea not to your liking at first. However, liking green tea can be learned. And if you just stick to it for the first few cups, you will eventually find yourself loving the refreshing light taste of green tea.

To help make yourself like tea, you can add other things to your tea to make it just to your liking. Adding fresh milk to a cup of warm green tea is always a good idea. If you like it to be sweet, why not add a couple of teaspoons of brown sugar or honey? The more cups of tea your drink a day, the better. So you might want to train yourself to start liking it early. Soon enough, you'll be surprised to find yourself looking for green tea in the afternoons or with your morning paper.

**Eat a Few Raw Garlic Cloves**

Garlic has wonderful anti-bacterial properties that can help in removing the toxins in your body that may be causing the imbalance that is making you break out.

Garlic is a very powerful antioxidant too. And so if you can tolerate the taste and the smell, try and chew and few cloves of garlic every day.

Start with just one and then slowly increase your intake. However, be careful when eating raw garlic cloves, because they can make your stomach burn and give you a bad breath when eaten on an empty stomach. So to make things easier, incorporate the raw garlic in your meal or simply eat it right after a good meal.

This is great to ward off the flu and colds as well because it boosts your immune systems. And it works like a dream and significantly decrease the appearance of pimples when you start ingesting raw consistently. Never forget to brush your teeth after chewing down some garlic cloves, or else your friends will be wondering what you ate for lunch.

**Egg White and Milk Face Mask**

Sounds like something you would use to make dessert, doesn't it? Well, you can also use it to make your skin look as sweet as dessert. Egg white has great skin tightening properties while milk contains lactic acid that works wonders to reveal softer, smoother skin.

**How to Use It:** To prepare this face mask, crack one end of an egg and let the egg white out into a clean bowl. Add about a tablespoon of powdered full cream milk. Whisk the mixture until the two ingredients have been completely mixed together. It will become a creamy-looking substance.

If you don't want to use your fingers, you can use an old but clean make-up brush to apply the mask to your face. Apply the mixture all over your face, except the areas around your eyes. Leave it on your face until the mask has dried. But if you want, you can leave it longer on. To rinse, wash your face with warm water. Make sure that you do not leave any residue of the mask on your face.

If you have still some of the mixture left, simply put transfer the leftover in a container that has a lid and keep it in the fridge for the next time that you need to apply this face mask again.

Because of the gentle ingredients of this face mask, you can put it on as often as you want; in fact, you can apply it daily for better results. This is a great mask to use for people who have acne-prone skin or who are struggling to get rid of the marks that are left behind by pimple breakouts.

# Chapter 7:
## A New You

If you follow the tips that have been elaborated so far in this book, then you will eventually start to see a big difference not only in the appearance of your skin but even in the way you feel about your health, your sleep, and your diet.

The whole goal is to not to transform you in order to make you a different person, but to restore you to the best you that you can be. These tips are of course not the end all be all in the natural approach to dealing with skin problems and achieving beautiful skin. There are probably hundreds of other skin tips that you will eventually come up with your own, as you begin to love taking advantage of natural and organic methods of achieving the perfect skin.

Hopefully, this book has helped you greatly in looking for the cure that you have always been looking for. It is important to point out that none of the previously mentioned tips, suggestions, and routines provide immediate and instant solutions to the skin problems that you may currently be struggling with. But they are proven and tested methods that though might take some time are 100 percent natural and more than capable of providing long-term positive results than most chemically formulated drugs and topical medications.

By the time that you have tried and seen for your-self the tips that are explained here, you should start looking into the mirror and seeing a new you, a more beautiful, more glowing, happier you, who is more confident to go out there into the world.

To maintain the positive results that you get from these natural remedies and solutions, it is necessary that you stick with your routine and make sure that you allow yourself to get adjust to it. Learn how to read how your skin reacts and respond accordingly.

The moment you notice that something is not working for you or is not giving you the results that it is supposed to produce, ditch it for a better solution. Our skin works better with something that it has gotten used to already. So the moment you strike upon the right regimen, stick with it and enjoy the results!

# Closing

Thank you for picking up this book and reading this far. But more than that, you should thank yourself for making the decision to take control of whatever condition your skin is in and choosing to make things better for yourself.

This book is no magic wand that will make all your skin-related worries go away, but it is definitely my aim to help you come upon a holistic regimen that will work like a miracle for you. And of course, the aim of this book is to help you give more importance to your skin, take better care of your health, and know for a fact that however bad the condition your skin may be in right now, it will get better. Things are bound to look up. You'll see.

What's important is that even after finishing reading this book, you would continue to be on the quest for more and better organic alternatives for beauty products and treatments that are very common today and to continue to value your health in such a way as to encourage you to never fail to pursue the healthy lifestyle.

Lastly, if this book has helped you in any way, you can share what tips you have learned here with others and help them uncover their most beautiful selves as well!